Macular Placque.

CANINE

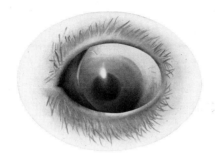

OPHTHALMOLOGY

William G. Magrane, D.V.M., M.Sc. (Med.)

Practitioner and Lecturer, specializing in diseases and surgery of the eye, Mishawaka, Indiana; Veterinary Ophthalmologist to the Division of Biology and Medicine, Atomic Energy Commission, Washington, D. C.; American Editor, British Journal of Small Animal Practice, London, England; Consulting Editor, Small Animal Clinician, Bonner Springs, Kansas; Consulting Editor, Animal Hospital, Journal of American Animal Hospital Association, Chicago, Illinois.

155 Figures with 224 Illustrations and
11 Color Plates, with 75 Illustrations

Lea & Febiger

Philadelphia

1965

Library of Congress Catalog Card Number 65–24803
Printed in the United States of America

This Book is Dedicated

to

my wife, Elaine

Who helped to make its writing possible

PREFACE

In this book I have endeavored to present a concise, practical, and systematic review of the diseases and surgical procedures of the canine eye. The text is intended for the student and general practitioner in veterinary medicine and includes principles of ophthalmology applicable to any of the species.

To remain within the scope of a manual, excessive detail, extensive discussion, theories and rare conditions are allotted minimal space. It is hoped that the reader will seek further knowledge in the subject by references to the more exhaustive and comprehensive textbooks of human ophthalmology. However, since some important differences do exist between the canine and human eye, a comparison will be made as deemed necessary.

There has been no attempt made to categorize all of the preparations and drugs or surgical procedures, nor to describe all methods of treatment or operative techniques. Only those with which I am most familiar are included.

Illustrations and photographs have been used when it seemed that they would be of value in clarifying the text. I am indebted to many colleagues in human and veterinary medicine for permission to use illustrative material and for their inspiration and help.

I wish to express my special appreciation to Denyes Studio of South Bend, Indiana, and Mr. James Sprunger in particular, illustrators for this book; and to my daughter-in-law Barbara, who typed and helped to edit the complete manuscript. I am deeply grateful to the many practitioners throughout the country who have provided me with the cases that have made this specialized study and this book possible.

William G. Magrane

CONTENTS

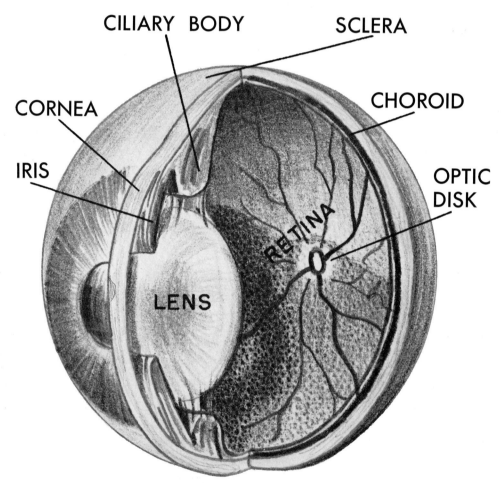

Fig. 1. The eye with section removed.

Chapter 1

THE NORMAL EYE

Vision

1:1   It is generally agreed that the domestic dog is myopic (near sighted), astigmatic (uneven cornea), color blind, and accommodates poorly. Roberts[1] concludes that the selection process which has produced dog breeds of greatly varying anatomical types has produced haphazard combinations of the various genetic factors that account for the optical system, the corneal size and shape, lens curvature, and anteroposterior measurements resulting in the poor visual apparatus of the dog breeds we know today. The dog has sharpened his other senses because his vision is so poor, at least when we compare it to man.

1:2   It has been determined by retinoscopy and ophthalmoscopy that the dog is uniformly myopic. This is to say that the eye is so constructed that the vision image comes to a focus in front of the retina (Fig. 2). We have noted degree variances of myopia from 1 to 8 diopters. The average, however, is about

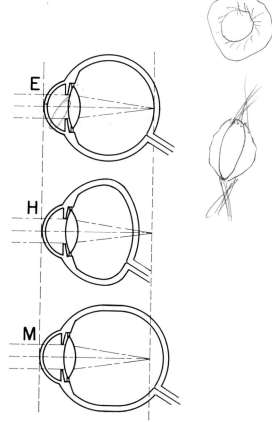

Fig. 2.   E, Emmetropia (normal sight). H, Hyperopia (far sighted). M, Myopia (near sighted).

9

3 diopters, and it is at a minus 3 setting that we initiate our ophthalmoscopic examination (Par. 2:50).

1:3   The poor accommodation (ability to focus) is the result of a weak ciliary muscle and a firm, well-implanted lens within the eye. This anatomical difference (*i.e.* from man) produces a naturally presbyopic eye (old sight) in the dog. In contrast, the eye of man does not ordinarily become presbyopic until middle age when the ciliary muscle loses its power and the lens becomes sclerotic.

1:4   For academic interest, a number of investigations[2] as to the color vision of the dog have been undertaken. The investigators have concluded: for the dog, it is form and (to a less extent) brightness which are important qualities of visual stimuli. It is doubtful if the animal experiences color at all. Whatever weakly chromatic sensations his cones may afford are further unsaturated and greatly diluted by his superabundant rods. That is, he sees shades of grey when looking at and comparing red and pink blankets.

1:5   Fortunately for the dog other factors play a role in providing satisfactory vision. He has a larger pupil and larger visual field than man, with a better peripheral vision. With the aid of the tapetum lucidum and abundant rods, the dog can see better in semi-darkened to darkened areas (Par. 11:15). He has a fair degree of binocular vision (depth perception), but whenever one eye is lost through disease or injury the other takes over in remarkable fashion, using a sense of perspective and parallactic displacement to compensate in part. On the whole, as is the case with all the species, the dog is supplied with the type of vision most suited to its needs, and is most adept in following moving objects.

1:6   The question often arises as to how long does it take after the eyes are open until the new puppy can see. Anatomically, the developmental processes of the eye itself are complete at birth, even though the lid junction does not disappear until approximately ten days postpartum. The time of lid opening, however, always coincides closely with that at which the rods and cones of the retina have finished their differentiation. We can only postulate as to when single binocular vision, with depth perception and fusion occurs. Based on an age comparison with man, this would be at about six weeks in the puppy.

Anatomy of Vision

1:7   The eye may be considered as an optical instrument comparable to the camera, in which by means of a refracting (dioptric) system a small and inverted image of external objects is formed on the retina.[3]

1:8   In passing through the eyeball rays of light traverse the cornea, aqueous, lens, and vitreous. These light rays are refracted (bent) to converge on or near the retina. The refracting surfaces of the eye are the cornea, and the anterior and posterior surfaces of the lens, although the cornea plays the principal role in this regard. The refracting media are the aqueous, lens substance, and the vitreous.

1:9   The amount of light is regulated by the eyelids and the pupillary action of the iris. Light reaching the retina is absorbed by its deeper layers and a photochemical reaction converts this light into nervous impulses. Nervous impulses arising here are transmitted in the reverse direction to the innermost retinal nerve fiber layer, and thence to the optic nerve. Impulses continue along the optic nerve, optic chiasm (where a partial decussation of fibers

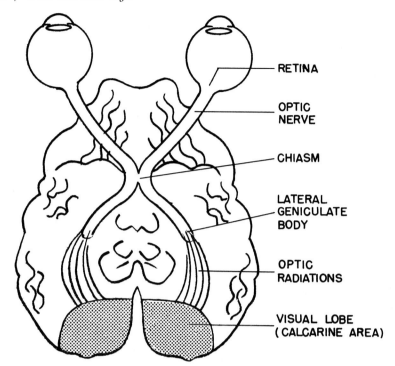

RETINA

OPTIC
NERVE

CHIASM

LATERAL
GENICULATE
BODY

OPTIC
RADIATIONS

VISUAL LOBE
(CALCARINE AREA)

Fig. 3.   The anatomy of vision.

takes place), optic tract, and into the lateral geniculate body. From the lateral geniculate body, optic radiations travel to the calcarine area of the occipital lobe of the cerebrum. It is here that impulses are recorded and interpreted (Fig. 3).

1:10   The eye, then, must not be considered an isolated organ, for the retina and all the refractive media are useless if the nerve connections to the cerebral cortex of the occipital lobe are diseased or cut off.[4]

Anatomy

General Considerations

1:11   The anatomical parts with which ophthalmology is concerned are the eyeball proper, the appendages of the eye, *i.e.* the cavity which contains the eye, the eyelids which protect it, the muscles which move it, the lacrimal apparatus which constantly moistens its

transparent portion, and the visual pathways just described (Par. 1:9).

1:12   This chapter will concern itself only with a view of the eyeball as a whole. The anatomy and physiology of each of the parts constituting the visual apparatus will be more precisely discussed at the beginning of the chapters dealing with the diseases and surgery of these parts.

1:13   Prince[5] describes the eye (Fig. 1) simply as a layer of neural light-sensitive tissue (the retina) held in shape by surrounding coats which protect it (sclera) and nourish it (choroid), and served by an optical system of a lens of modified transparent epithelium behind a transparent anterior extension of the sclera (cornea), all of which combine to focus light on the retina.

1:14   The eyeball proper consists of three layers or tunics:

1. *External fibrous tunic.* The outer protective layer which, with the intraocular pressure given the globe its definite semi-rigid shape. This layer could be likened to the box of a camera.

    a. Anterior portion: *Cornea*
    b. Posterior portion: *Sclera*

Both of these parts are covered by conjunctiva which is represented by epithelium only over the transparent cornea.

2. *Vascular tunic* (Uvea). This layer provides for the nourishment of the eyeball and is composed of:

    a. Iris
    b. Ciliary body (ciliary muscle and ciliary processes)
    c. Choroid

3. *Inner layer: Retina.* A thin, delicate membrane which is really an expansion of the optic nerve. All parts of the eye serve the purpose of protecting and maintaining the retina.

1:15   Within the eyeball are the principal structures referred to as:

1. The *anterior chamber* containing *aqueous* humor.
2. *Pupil*—formed by action of the iris.
3. *Posterior chamber*—containing aqueous and vitreous humor.
4. *Lens* and its *zonular* attachments.
5. *Vitreous* humor—a jelly-like mass occupying the greater part of the ocular

cavity and lying between the posterior surface of the lens and the retina. Its outer surface presents a thin, structureless condensation, the *hyaloid membrane,* which, in turn, is firmly attached to the posterior capsule of the lens.

1:16   External structures include:

Bulbar conjuctiva—covers the globe proper.

Palpebral conjunctiva—lines the upper and lower lids.

Limbus—the peripheral area 1 mm wide, which forms a transition zone between the cornea and the conjunctiva-sclera. It is rich in blood vessels and nerve endings like the conjunctiva.

Tenon's capsule—a dense connective tissue membrane which surrounds most of the eye and its muscles and is located between the bulbar conjunctiva and the underlying sclera.

Episclera—a thin, spongy, vascular, elastic membrane whose purpose is to provide nutrition to the outer parts of the almost avascular sclera. It is contained within Tenon's capsule and loosely attached to the globe by fibrous connective tissue.

1:17   *Extraocular muscles* (Fig. 4) are seven in number. There are four recti, two obliques and a retractor oculi (absent in man). The recti and obliques

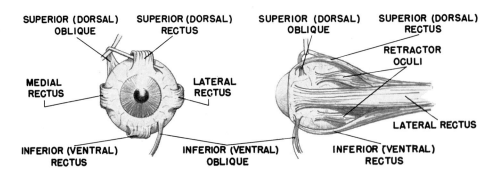

FRONT VIEW   LATERAL VIEW

Fig. 4.   The extraocular muscles.

are poorly developed as compared to man.

1:18   All four recti muscles are flat, have their origins around the optic foramen and orbital fissure and insert into the globe with aponeurotic tendons between 6 and 8 mm from the limbus.

1:19   The inferior and superior oblique muscles which serve as rotators of the eye in the dog are attached near the insertions of the recti in the anterior portion of the eye. This is in sharp contrast to man where these muscles insert posterior to the equator.

1:20   The retractor oculi may be either a complete cone of muscle, the apex at the orbital fissure and the base at its insertions into the globe, or it may be divided into four parts, two inserting on either side of the superior rectus and the other two on either side of the inferior rectus. The retractor oculi serves

a useful purpose in providing a protective mechanism for the eye. Since there is no complete bony orbit in the dog, it is important that the eye can be retracted in impending danger.

Measurements (Fig. 5.)

1:21   The eye is almost spherical and is relatively large for the size of the animal. The geometrical center of the cornea is known as the *anterior pole* of the eye and the *posterior pole* is exactly opposite and is usually dorsal and medial to the nerve head. The *geometric axis* connects the anterior and posterior poles.

1:22   There are three diameters which are commonly referred to as: the *sagittal* (anteroposterior), the *transverse* and the *vertical*. The length of these varies among the different breeds with a dimensional range of:

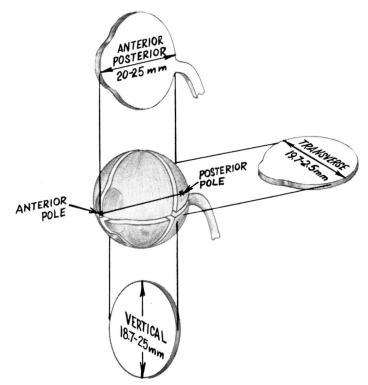

Fig. 5.   Measurements of the canine eye in the anteroposterior, transverse, and vertical directions.

20.0 to 25 mm in the anteroposterior direction

19.7 to 25 mm in the transverse direction

18.7 to 25 mm in the vertical direction

1:23   The total absolute volume of the eyeball is from 4.5 to 5 cc and the weight from 4 to 8 grams.

The Vascular System (Fig. 6)

1:24   The main blood supply to the orbit is derived from the internal maxillary artery, which is a continuation of the external carotid artery. Two branches of the internal maxillary artery penetrate the periorbita and represent the external ophthalmic artery.

1:25   The ciliary system is derived from the external ophthalmic artery and is distributed through the vascular tunic and sclera by:

(1) Four to six short posterior ciliary arteries which ramify within the choroid.

(2) Two long posterior ciliary arteries which run between the sclera and choroid and give off branches to the ciliary muscle, ciliary processes, and the iris.

(3) The anterior ciliary arteries which supply branches to the conjunctiva, sclera, ciliary muscles, and limbal region.

1:26   The venous tributaries converge towards the equator, perforate the sclera and pass into the ophthalmic vein. The anterior branches unite into an annular plexus which receives the veins of the ciliary body and iris. The anterior ciliary veins communicate with the *plexus venosus sclerae* (drainage system).

Nerve Supply (Fig. 7.)

1:27   The nerves of the eyeball course toward the cornea between the

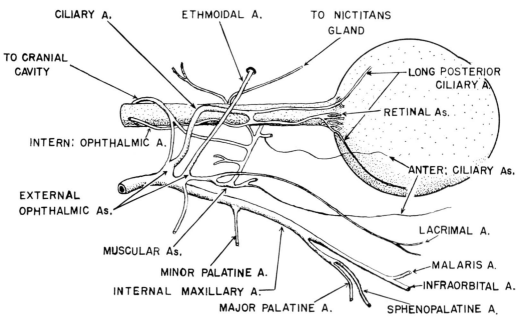

Fig. 6.   The orbital arterial system. (Prince, Diesem, Eglitis and Ruskell, *Anatomy and Histology of the Eye and Orbit in Domestic Animals,* courtesy of Charles C Thomas.)

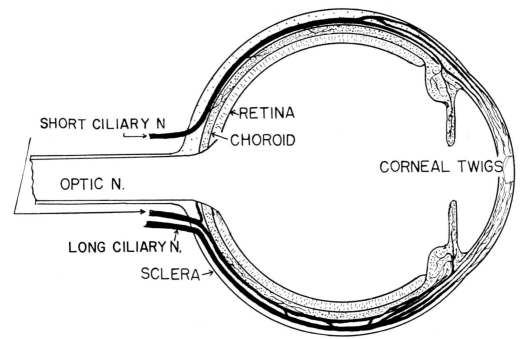

Fig. 7.   The paths by which the various ciliary nerves enter the eye, anastomose, and travel to their destinations. (Prince, Diesem, Eglitis and Ruskell, *Anatomy and Histology of the Eye and Orbit in Domestic Animals,* courtesy of Charles C Thomas.)

sclera and choroid and form a plexus in the choroid and then the plexus gangliosus ciliaris on the ciliary body, which gives rise to the nerves for the ciliary muscle, the iris, and the cornea.

General Nerve Supply

1:28   Third (Oculomotor) supplies motor fibers to: superior, inferior and medial recti muscles, portion of the retractor oculi, inferior oblique, levator, sphincter of iris, ciliary muscle.
Fourth (Trochlear) supplies the superior oblique.
Fifth (Ophthalmic branch of trigeminal) supplies: lids, conjunction, cornea, dilators of the iris.
Sixth (Abducens) supplies the lateral rectus and portions of the retractor oculi.
Seventh (Facial) supplies the orbicularis muscle.

For a more comprehensive study of the neurology the reader is referred to the texts mentioned in the references.

References

1. Roberts, S. R.: Animal Vision, J.A.V.M.A., *127,* 236, 1955.
2. Walls, Gordon L.: *The Vertebrate Eye,* Bloomfield Hills, Cranbrook Institute of Science, p. 506, 1942.
3. Allen, James H.: *May's Diseases of the Eye,* 23rd ed., Baltimore, The Williams & Wilkins Co., 1963.
4. Leinfelder, P. J.: Outline of Neuro-ophthalmology, Home Study Course, Am. Ac. Ophth. & Otolar.
5. Prince, Jack H., Diesem, Charles D., Eglitis, Irma and Ruskell, Gordon L.: *Anatomy and Histology of the Eye and Orbit in Domestic Animals,* Springfield, Charles C Thomas, 1960.
6. Cello, Robert M., Krawitz, Leonard and Magrane, William G.: Anatomy Notes, Home Study Course, Am. Soc. Vet. Ophthal.
7. Trautmann, Alfred and Fiebiger, Josef: *Fundamentals of the Histology of Domestic Animals,* 8th and 9th ed., Ithaca, Comstock Publishing Associates, 1952.

Chapter 2

EXAMINATION OF THE EYE AND ITS ADNEXA

External Examination

2:1   The clinician must ever remember that ophthalmology is a branch of medicine and surgery. Examination of an eye or eyes does not mean merely that an isolated organ is being studied, rather, that the animal is being examined with special reference to that organ and its functions. It is often imperative that an accurate case history, thorough physical examination, and laboratory studies are necessary before an evaluation of the ocular lesion is possible.

2:2   Every examination should include a systematic plan, a routine that will enable the examiner mentally to catalogue his findings in orderly fashion and instill in him the concept of thinking of the eyeball and adnexa as a whole. Unless this principal is adhered to, an obvious lesion of one part of the globe will often distract the examiner so that either the real cause of that lesion or associated pathologic condition is completely overlooked.

2:3   Examination of the eye may be divided into: (1) objective and (2) subjective (functional).

2:4   The objective examination consists first of a naked eye examination of the dog. This procedure is applicable primarily to the orbit and eyelids. It is conducted with *minimal restraint* being used and is for the purpose of ascertaining obvious abnormalities such as swellings, comparing size of the eyes, discharges, size of the palpebral aperture, and especially the position of the lids in relation to the globe. It may be necessary to withold all restraint and examine the patient on the floor in

16

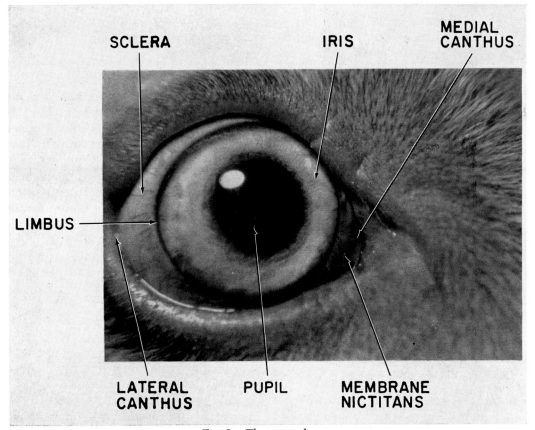

SCLERA   IRIS   MEDIAL CANTHUS

LIMBUS

LATERAL CANTHUS   PUPIL   MEMBRANE NICTITANS

Fig. 8. The external eye.

order to determine accurately the lid relationship (*e.g.* entropion, ectropion) to the globe.

2:5 For the remainder of the objective examination I feel that this can be properly conducted only in a semi-darkened to dark room with the aid of proper equipment and suitable, focal light source. A binocular magnifier of some type and a light source, *e.g.* a pen-light, will, in most instances, suffice to examine properly all structures to and including the lens (Fig. 9). A hand (portable) "slit"-lamp (Fig. 10) will offer a more detailed and magnified view of these same structures as will the ophthalmoscope with the proper lens setting (Par. 2:50). The hand type

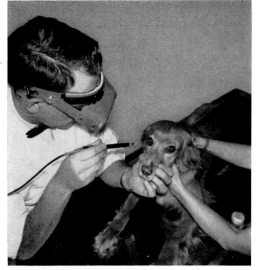

Fig. 9. Examination of the eye utilizing a binocular loupe and focal light source (darkened room essential).

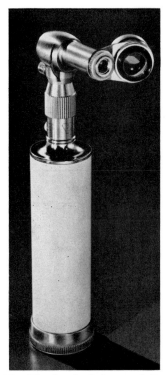

Fig. 10. The hand slit-lamp of Bausch and Lomb.

slit-lamp is relatively inexpensive and practical for use, and is not to be confused with the giant, stationary type (Par. 2:6) (Fig. 11).

2:6   Überreiter[1] has pioneered in the use of biomicroscopy for examination of the eye in animals. The combination of the corneal microscope with illumination by a slit-lamp for the examination of the anterior portion of the eye offers a magnification of 10 to 60 diameters and enables the viewer to observe finer structures and localize the depth of pathologic processes. This piece of equipment is essential to the specialist in human or animal ophthalmology, but because of the cost factor and need for special training in its use, is not practical for general use. Various slit-lamp models may be modified for use by the veterinary ophthalmologist. With the aid of simple tranquilization a thorough examination can then be conducted (Fig. 11). On occasion it has proven to be the *only* means of arriving at a correct diagnosis with subsequent correction of a chronic condition.

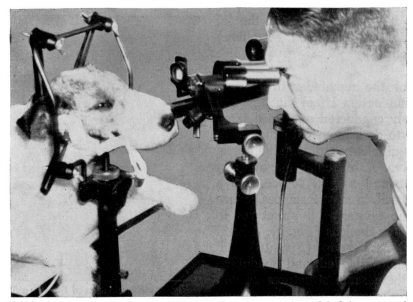

Fig. 11. The slit-lamp and corneal microscope (biomicroscopy) modified for use in the dog.

2:7 *Transillumination* is useful when corneal edema and/or flocculent debris in the anterior chamber precludes examination of the iris and pupillary area.[2] Often even the lens and vitreal cavity can be visualized by this means. This method of examination uses the passage of a beam of light through the sclera. The light source is applied directly to the globe at different aspects of the sclera, usually near the limbus. Good results can only be obtained when the examining room is absolutely dark.

2:8 Various types of transilluminators are used. Ophthalmoscopes can be adapted for this purpose (Fig. 12). Small pen-lights and varied diagnostic equipment with intense focal light source will also serve the purpose.

2:9 *Gonioscopy*—The angle of the anterior chamber (iris angle) is hidden from view in man and animals by the forward projection of the opaque edge of the scleral limbus. None of the ordinary methods of examination of the iris and chamber can reach this recess. Gonioscopy involves the observation of this angle of the anterior chamber of the living eye.

2:10 Whereas visualization of the chamber angle is desirable for other reasons, *e.g.* tumors, cysts, congenital anomalies, foreign bodies, the most important aspect of gonioscopy is in the study of glaucoma (Par. 9:51). Since certain tissues in the angle area are important in returning the aqueous humor to the blood stream, changes in these tissues can cause inhibition of outflow and give rise to an increase in intraocular pressure (Chapter 9). Study of the angle may reveal both cause and effect of glaucoma, and by so doing may furnish clues for medical or surgical treatment.

2:11 Gonioscopy in the dog is not particularly difficult to perform and has proven to be a most practical clinical procedure, although, admittedly its use is limited to the clinician who tends towards specialization.

2:12 Troncoso[13] gives a splendid word picture and color drawing of the canine chamber angle. One of several special contact glasses is placed upon the cornea and then by using strong illumination in combination with magnification (loupe, otoscope head, ophthalmoscope, or slit-lamp head) the angle can be studied[12].

Specific Structures

2:13 To begin the gross examination, it is necessary that the eye be cleansed when serous or purulent secretions obscure the globe and membranes (Par. 3:9). However, since it is often advantageous to take a swab for bacteriological and sensitivity studies, these tests should be anticipated before the irrigation and cleansing process is initiated.

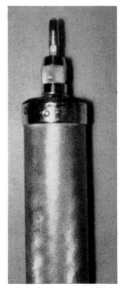

Fig. 12. Ophthalmoscope adapted for transillumination by removing the head.

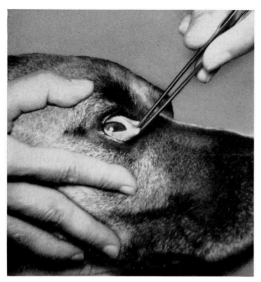

Fig. 13. Use of thumb forceps for examination of the membrane nictitans.

2:14   *Lids:* Note their thickness and position (entropion, ectropion); condition of their margin, whether swollen, crusted or ulcerated; presence of neoplasms; size of the opening; ability to open and close; openings for the lacrimal drainage system; presence of misdirected or a second row of cilia. The conjunctival surface (palpebral conjunctiva) is next inspected, especially if the presence of a foreign body is suspected. Exposure of the conjunctiva of the lower lid is easily accomplished by placing a finger near the margin of the lid and pressing downward. Eversion of the upper lid for viewing of the inner surface is more difficult but can be accomplished by grasping the center, pulling away from the globe and then back and upwards. A topical anesthetic (Par. 3:37) may be helpful or essential to the proper examination of this structure, the bulbar conjunctiva, and the cornea.

2:15   *Globe* proper: Note its situation in the orbit (exophthalmos, enophthalmos), mobility as compared to the companion eye and the presence of nystagmus.

2:16   *Conjunctiva*—bulbar: observe whether there is any edema (chemosis), signs of anemia, congestion, follicles, hyperplasia, growths, rents, or unusual amount of pigment deposition. Note possible presence of any foreign bodies, especially in the area of the *fornix* (upper transition of palpebral to bulbar conjunctiva), or in the *cul-de-sac* (lower transition of palpebral to bulbar conjunctiva).

2:17   *Membrane Nictitans:* This structure is a cartilaginous extension of the bulbar conjunctiva and is best examined under topical anesthesia. The superior border is grasped with smooth thumb forceps (Fig. 13), pulled up and out for a good view of the inner lymphoid surface and straight up to best see the external surface and conjunctival cul-de-sac. Note possible presence of follicles on either surface and especially for foreign bodies (*e.g.* weed seeds, etc.) between the inner surface and the globe.

2:18   *Lacrimal Drainage Apparatus:* It is often necessary to determine the

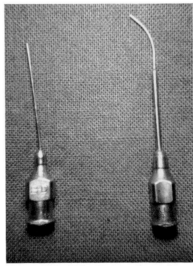

Fig. 14. Lacrimal canula.

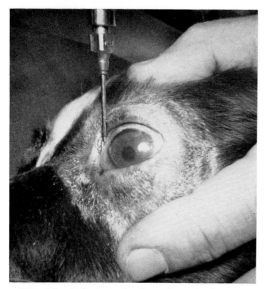

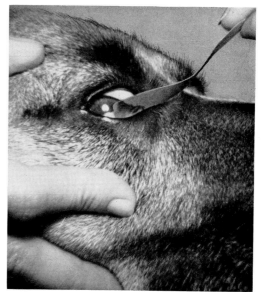

Fig. 15. Infusion of saline through the upper canaliculi to determine patency of the lacrimal drainage apparatus.

Fig. 17. Use of sterile fluorescein impregnated papers.

patency of the tear conducting channels to their nasal termination. This is easily accomplished under topical anesthesia and/or tranquilizers by introducing a blunt lacrimal canula (Fig. 14) into either the upper or lower slit-like openings (punctum) of the lacrimal canal and infusing saline solution (Fig. 15). When the drainage system is functioning properly, the solution will escape freely through the other duct opening and through the nostril. Entry and flushing is most easily accomplished through the upper opening. For probing the canals, various whalebone or metal bougies may be employed (Fig. 16).

2:19   *Cornea:* The cornea is normally clear, transparent and there should be no visible blood vessels. Note for pres-

ence of dullness, opacities, vascularization, foreign bodies, growths, conjunctival encroachment, pigmentation, and whether the surface is smooth and curved properly. To bring an abrasion or ulceration into view, fluorescein impregnated papers (Par. 3:68) are inserted in the lower cul-de-sac long enough to transfer the stain to the anterior aspect of the globe (Fig. 17). The excess is rinsed away with the wash bottle.

2:20   The sensitiveness of the cornea may be noted by touching it with a wisp of cotton, thread, or glass rod. The head of the dog should be held in such a position as to eliminate squinting caused by discomfort.

2:21   If deep ulceration and an im-

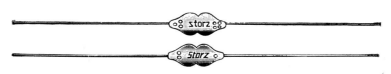

Fig. 16.   Metal probes (Bowman) used for probing the lacrimal canals

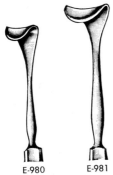

E-980   E-981
Fig. 18.   Lid retractor.

pending prolapse is evident, the examination is stopped immediately and adequate sedation administered. At the appropriate time following sedation, a general intravenous anesthesia is administered, the examination concluded, and, if possible, corrective measures are taken, thus eliminating the danger of anterior chamber rupture caused by undue restraint and activity on the part of the patient.

2:22   Lid retractors (Fig. 18) may be helpful in separating the lids for a better view of the cornea, especially when spasm of the lids (blepharospasm) prevents a proper examination. In every instance of this sort a topical anesthetic must be employed.

2:23   *Sclera:* The sclera is best examined by opening the palpebral fissure as widely as possible with the fingers or lid retractors and by changing the head position. This structure should be white and glistening underneath its covering of bulbar conjunctiva. Note the possible presence of subconjunctival hemorrhage (ecchymosis), episcleral injection and congestion, growths, embedded foreign bodies or the site of their entry into the globe, and jaundiced discoloration.

2:24   *Anterior Chamber:* Note its depth, whether normal, shallow, or increased; comparing it with the other eye when possible. The depth is apt to be shallow in glaucoma. The aqueous humor should be clear. If altered, observe whether there is a diffuse cloudiness (aqueous flare) or exudates consisting of pus (hypopyon) or blood (hyphema). Both direct and lateral illumination should be used.

2:25   *Iris:* The iris should be examined with both direct and lateral illumination. Observe its color, smoothness and texture, and whether it is steady or tremulous during movements of the eyeball (iridodenesis). The latter condition is seen when the iris is not properly supported by the anterior aspect of the lens, *e.g.* in absence (aphakia), subluxation, or luxation of the lens (Par. 9:67). Note especially whether there are adhesions to the cornea (anterior synechia) or to the anterior capsule of the lens (posterior synechia) and for atrophic changes of particularly the pupillary border.

2:26   *Pupil:* (Par. 7:13–7:19) Note its size, shape, position, compare its size with that of the other eye and especially its reaction to light stimuli. The normal pupil dilates when the eye is covered or in the dark and contracts when exposed to light. Both pupils should be equal in size under the same light conditions. In apprehensive dogs placed on the examining table, it will often be noted that the pupils react sluggishly to light stimuli. In these instances we also check the pupillary response out of doors, with the animal on the ground or comforted in the owner's arms.

2:27   *Lens:* Immediately behind the pupil the central aspect of the lens will be readily visible. Note for the presence of intralenticular opacities, and uveal pigment deposits on the anterior capsule. To explore the lens fully, dilatation of the pupil is necessary (Par.

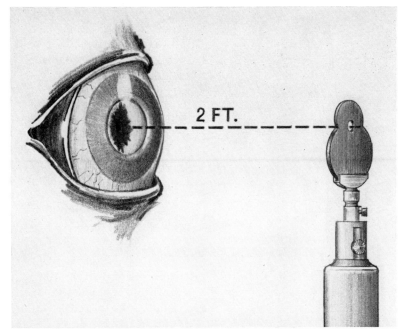

Fig. 19. Examination of the lens with the ophthalmoscope held at a distance.

2:44). In the aging dog a gray reflex (nuclear sclerosis) (Par. 10:28), must be expected and allowed for. An accurate evaluation of the lens can be accomplished by examining at a distance of 2 to 3 feet in a dark room with a pen-light or the 0 lens of the ophthalmoscope. The fundic reflex will serve as a background for the discerning of lens opacities (Fig. 19). Or, a close-up evaluation can be made with the plus 6–12 lens of the ophthalmoscope (Par. 2:50).

Palpation and Tension Determination

2:28   To complete the external examination, palpation is helpful in determining the presence or absence of pain in the ciliary region and for the existence of tumors and swellings in and around the orbit.

2:29   With practice, a fairly accurate approximation of intraocular tension can also be achieved by digital palpation. With the two index fingers placed upon the upper lid, the globe is pal-

pated by an alternating rolling motion of the fingers (Fig. 20). Some idea of the degree of tension may then be determined by comparison with the other eye, if normal, or with another healthy eye.

2:30   For accurate determination of intraocular pressure, an instrument known as the tonometer must be used (Fig. 21). It records resistance offered

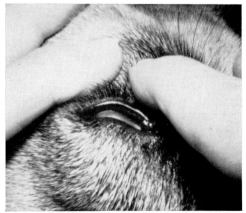

Fig. 20. Testing the tension of the eyeball by digital tonometry.

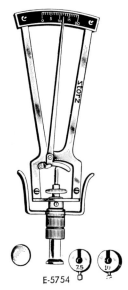

Fig. 21. Schiötz tonometer.

to definite weights used to produce an indentation of the cornea, by movement of a needle upon a scale. While used routinely in human ophthalmology, it has not been generally adopted by the veterinarian, although it most certainly has a place in the resources of the small-animal practitioner who interests himself in diseases and surgery of the eye.[6]

2:31　　The tonometer has been found especially useful; (1) in the early diagnosis of glaucoma, with suspected alteration in tension, (2) following surgical procedures or medicinal treatment for the correction of glaucoma, and (3) for keeping a "check" on the unaffected eye in glaucoma patients.[12]

2:32　　The tonometer in general use is the model of Schiötz. In cooperative patients, readings can be made following two instillations of a topical anesthetic, five minutes being allowed to elapse between instillations. An assistant restrains the animal's head in such manner that the eyes are directed upwards, the lids are separated, and the tonometer is allowed to rest by its own

weight upon the near center of the upturned cornea (Fig. 22). In puppies and dogs with small eyes, it is difficult to take accurate readings because of the size of the cup at the base of the instrument.

2:33　　Normal intraocular pressure in the dog varies between 16 and 30 mm Hg with the average between 20 and 25 mm Hg. This corresponds with the normal pressure of the eye in man.

Subjective Examination

2:34　　Subjective or functional examination of the eye is, of course, difficult in dumb animals. A true evaluation of pain, light and dark adaptation, field of vision, and percentage of vision is impossible. Veterinary clinicians then should not be guilty of assuring the client that his pet has, let us say, 25 per cent vision in the right eye and 75 per cent in the left.

2:35　　However, much can be learned by eliciting a good history as regards movement of the dog throughout the house, up and down lighted and unlighted stairs, out of doors on dark versus sunlit days, reaction to large versus

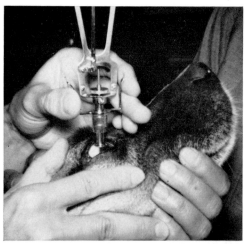

Fig. 22.　Testing the tension of the eyeball by instrumental tonometry.

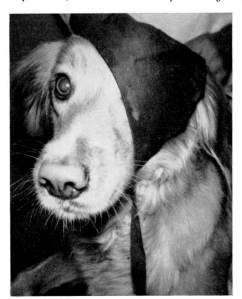

Fig. 23. Black patch with ties used to test the vision of the fellow eye.

small objects, reaction to changes in furniture placement, ability to jump on sofas and beds, follow rolling balls, and finding tidbits held up or thrown. Pain is shown by rubbing of the affected side on the rug, furniture or owner's leg and often by a change in disposition, eating habits, and general lethargy.

2:36 Patching of the unaffected eye (Fig. 23) and subjecting the dog to an obstacle course around the examining room will also be of value in vision determination. The clinician and owner should remain stationary while this test is being conducted.

2:37 Finally, the clinician is cautioned about using the "hand waving technique" for vision determination. Air currents created by this motion cause lid blinking and globe reaction which are not indications of sight perception.

Internal Examination (Ophthalmoscopy)

2:38 When the ocular media is sufficiently clear, the deeper internal structures, *i.e.* vitreous humor and fundus, are examined with an ophthalmoscope. Ophthalmoscopy has been recognized as a valuable addition to medical diagnostic procedures for over a hundred years. Its use has been limited in veterinary medicine primarily because of insufficient training and lack of emphasis of its importance. The ophthalmoscope, when used properly and frequently, becomes a most useful diagnostic tool for the determination of ocular fundic degenerations and lesions, injuries, congenital anomalies, growths, and even certain systemic diseases (Chapter 12). In addition, by utilizing the plus lens system, all parts of the eye from the cornea through the vitreous can be studied with this instrument (Fig. 24).

2:39 There are two general methods of ophthalmoscopic examination: direct and indirect. The indirect method utilizes a condensing lens between the patient's eye and the ophthalmoscope. The more modern equipment of this type is very expensive, has a lower magnifying capacity, and cannot be used to examine the more anterior portions of the globe. Its chief usefulness is in specialty work and research where it is used to examine the more peripheral fundus.[7]

2:40 It is with the direct method which we are concerned. In the direct method a beam of light is thrown into the interior of the patient's eye by a reflector, while the aperture in the lens-disc, which opening is situated above the level of the reflector, allows a portion of this light, after returning from the patient's eye, to pass into the eye of the observer. This method utilizes the common electric ophthalmoscope.[8]

2:41 In initiating the examination

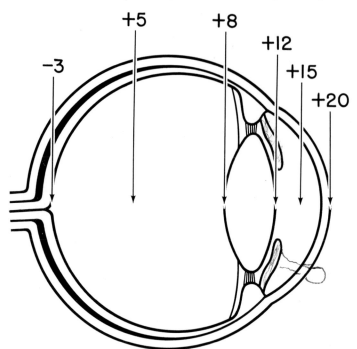

Fig. 24. With the ophthalmoscope 1 inch in front of the eye, the lens in the rotating wheel produce clear vision at points indicated in the diagrammatic eye.

with the ophthalmoscope, it is often useful to hold the instrument at a distance of about 2 feet (Par. 2:27). At this distance and with the 0 setting, one is better able to detect lesions, especially of the lens, that may be missed when the instrument is held close to the eye.

2:42 The clinician with a refractive error of his own may choose to wear his glasses or not when using the ophthalmoscope. If, however, this refractive error is marked and he chooses not to wear glasses for the examination, the difference should be taken into consideration. For example, hyperopia of one's eye will tend to neutralize myopia of the patient's (Par. 1:2).

Suggestions for Using the Ophthalmoscope

2:43 1. The examination should be performed in a well darkened room, and where distracting influences are minimal. One of the deterrents to the successful use of this instrument is the lack of cooperation of the patient. This is seldom a problem if the dog is restrained comfortably in a quiet room with only the owner, assistant and observer present. It is well to have the owner stand where the dog can see and be reassured of his presence.

2:44 2. Dilatation of the pupil is not always necessary, but it is helpful to the novice, and is advisable if the periphery of the fundus is to be examined. In pathological dilatation (Par. 11:49) this, of course, will not be necessary. Agents which may be used for dilatation include Mydricyl, Neosynephrine, or Cyclogyl (Par. 3:30). Several instillations are made over a thirty-minute period. These mydriatrics lose their effect within a few hours.

2:45 3. The owner or assistant may satisfactorily restrain the animal's head.

Obviously, however, a trained assistant is preferable for this purpose.

2:46 4. The head of the ophthalmoscope should be held about 1 inch away from the patient's cornea. Both eyes should be examined. When examining the right eye, the observer uses his right eye and sits or stands on the right side. When examining the left eye, the observer must be to the left and use his left eye. If, however, the habit of using only one eye for the examination has already been established, it is not important that this routine be changed.

2:47 5. The ophthalmoscope is held vertically (Fig. 25) in front of the observer's eye with the light beam directed toward the patient, and the right index finger is placed on the serrated edge of the dial in order to change lenses as necessary. The observer will soon learn to follow the natural movement of the dog's eye or, it may be advantageous to remain fixed, thus allowing the movements to bring the different aspects of the fundus into view.

2:48 6. In looking through the ophthalmoscope the observer should relax his accommodation and gaze through the eye, not at the eye, *i.e.* across the fields into the distant horizon. The observer's other eye may be suppressed without closing, in the manner of using a monocular microscope.

2:49 One of the most troublesome barriers to a good view of the fundus is the light reflected back into the examiner's eye by the patient's cornea. Two methods may be used to minimize this nuisance. The first is to use the pin hole aperture. However, this method reduces the area illuminated. The second is to direct the light beam toward the edge of the pupil rather than directly through the center. A little practice with this method is soon rewarded by much better views of the fundus.

2:50 7. Since most dogs are myopic (Par. 1:2), the minus 3 lens is first used to focus on the optic disc and retina. By changing the lens to more or less minus, the fundus is brought into the clearest view for the observer. Ophthalmoscopy is also a means of determining the approximate degree of myopia, or hyperopia (if the plus lens system must be used). Then by rotation from the minus through the plus lens the structures anterior to the fundus may be brought into view (Fig. 24). Vitreous opacities may be picked up between 0 and plus 6–8; the lens between plus 6–8 and plus 12, thence through the plus lens to the iris, anterior chamber, and the cornea itself, which is in position at about plus 20.

2:51 8. Patience and precise observations are necessary for obtaining diagnostic information, and thorough familiarity with the normal structure of

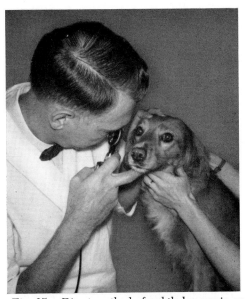

Fig. 25. Direct method of ophthalmoscopic examination.

the eye is necessary before disease processes can be recognized. This is especially true of the dog's eye in which there are many variations of the normal.[9]

2:52   Familiarity with the normal can only be achieved by using the ophthalmoscope at every opportunity. Its routine use in the general physical examination of a patient will soon result in a surprising acumen and will, in addition, often prove of value in assaying a systemic condition (Chapter 12).

Fundus and Retina of the Adult Dog (after H. B. Parry)[10]

2:53   The fundus of the dog differs from that of man in the presence of a tapetum lucidum and a heavily pigmented choroid, as well as in the absence of a true macula or fovea. This area in the dog is known as the *area centralis.*

2:54   The fundus can be divided conveniently into two portions: (Plate 1A)
1. The tapetal fundus in the dorsal quadrants backed by the brightly reflecting tapetum lucidum.
2. The non-tapetal fundus (tapetum nigrum) dark with choroidal pigment in the ventral quadrants.
The tapetal fundus is half-moon shaped, occupying most of the dorsal quadrants, but *not* extending to the periphery of the fundus, where it is surrounded by a narrow zone of non-tapetal fundus.

2:55   The color of the tapetum lucidum varies from a light lemon yellow through orange to a deep apple green, dependent upon the breed and the individual. In some breeds, such as pointers, the color of the reflection appears to be inherited with certain coat colors (*e.g.* liver coat color and a light orange brown tapetum), but in most breeds this association is not very distinct.

2:56   Over the tapetal fundus, the retina appears to be fully translucent without refractive distortion and its surface is flat, but the substance of the fundus appears to have a definite texture of fine granular beading, which becomes slightly coarser towards the periphery. Between the beading is a very fine reticulum of dark triangular spaces, the stellulae of Winslow. The granular beading is most marked in adolescent dogs; in some animals over two years old the texture of the granular beading is so fine that it appears to be even.

2:57   A single group of primary dorsal retinal blood vessels arises from the central retinal artery and vein and passes dorsally from the disc, where it gives rise to numerous secondary branches which ramify upwards and outwards as sharply defined thin-walled vessels lying on or just within the surface layers of the retina. The area centralis is only detectable by a slight reduction in the density of the secondary blood vessels over a portion of the tapetal fundus, dorsal and temporal to the disc. At the periphery of the tapetal fundus, the tapetum becomes irregular with areas of dark non-tapetal fundus interposed; occasionally similar areas

---

Plate 1.
    A. Fundus drawing. Adult dog.
    B. Fundus photograph. Normal disc and tapetum lucidum. Courtesy: Dr. F. Lescure, de l'Ecole Nationale Vëterinaire de Toulouse.
    C. Fundus photograph. Normal disc embedded in tapetum nigrum.

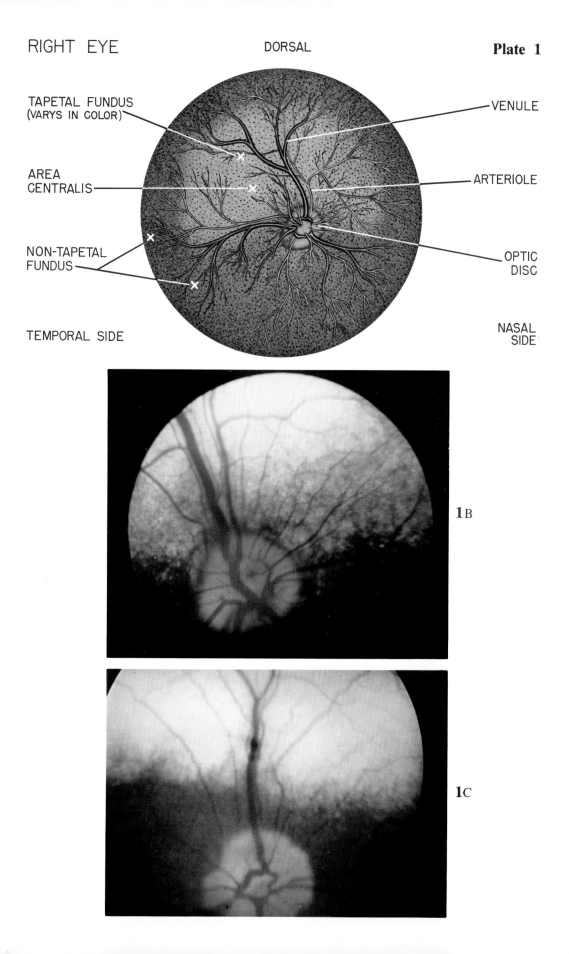

RIGHT EYE

DORSAL

Plate 1

TAPETAL FUNDUS
(VARYS IN COLOR)

VENULE

AREA
CENTRALIS

ARTERIOLE

NON-TAPETAL
FUNDUS

OPTIC
DISC

TEMPORAL SIDE

NASAL
SIDE

1B

1C

free of tapetum occur in the mid-tapetal fundus.

2:58 The non-tapetal fundus is a deep brown color, due to the choroidal pigment, with a slight grey over-wash. The granular texture is not so well marked in this region. The blood vessels arising from the two main medial and lateral horizontal retinal vessels are more numerous over the ventral non-tapetal fundus than over the tapetal fundus and the larger vessels reflect the light from their surface, producing a thin regular "silver-wire" reflection, which is not seen with the tapetal vessels.

2:59 The optic papilla (disc) usually lies just within the ventral border of the tapetal fundus not infrequently surrounded by a narrow zone of non-tapetal fundus. It is situated nasally from the center and is round to oval. Its margins are well demarcated in some dogs and ragged in others. There are three main groups of blood vessels, the dorsal and the two horizontal, medial and lateral. The venous vessels usually arise from a circular vessel connected to the central retinal vein, while the three arterial vessels arise independently in the substance of the papilla near its center. The venules are larger and darker than the arterials. At the junction of the peripheral and central portions of the papilla, some ten to fifteen small subsidiary arterial vessels arise within the substance of the papilla and run radially outwards over the peripapillary retina. Usually the papilla (disc) is flat with its periphery level with the inner surface of the retina, although in about one-third there will be evident a physiological pit 1–2 diopters deep. The papilla is usually pinkish white.

2:60 Observation of the choroid, other than the tapetum, is restricted to the dense brown pigment in its inner layers over the non-tapetal fundus. The pigment completely obscures the choroidal blood vessels in most normal dogs, although it is possible to view the choroidal circulation in many light coated dogs. (Plate 11*H*)

2:61 Szutter[11] has described the development of eye-background coloring in the puppy two weeks until the fourth month of age. The colors most often seen in the tapetum lucidum were greenish yellow, yellow-gold, and bright green. During the development of the colors the most consistent intermediate color was lilac. In the tapetum nigrum (non-tapetal fundus) the commonly seen colors were: rust red, yellowish brown, greenish brown, and brownish-black. From the time the eyelids opened until the thirtieth day, the overall color of the eye background appeared bluish-grey.

References

1. Überreiter, Von Otto: Examination of the Eye and Eye Operations in Animals, *Advances in Veterinary Science*, Vol. 5, New York, Academic Press, Inc., 1959.
2. Allen, James H.: *May's Diseases of the Eye*, 23rd ed., Baltimore, The Williams & Wilkins Co., 1963.
3. Selinger, Elias: *Office Treatment of the Eye*, Chicago, The Year Book Publishers, Inc., 1949.
4. Rutherford, C. W.: *The Eye*, New York, D. Appleton & Co., 1929.
5. Adler, Francis H.: *Gifford's Textbook of Ophthalmology*, 7th ed., Philadelphia, W. B. Saunders Co., 1962.
6. Magrane, William G.: Tonometry in Ophthalmology, No. Am. Vet., *32*, 413, 1951.
7. Rubin, L. F.: Indirect Ophthalmoscopy in Veterinary Medicine, J.A.V.M.A., *137*, 648, 1960.
8. Catcott, Earl J.: Ophthalmoscopy in Canine Practice, J.A.V.M.A., *121*, 35, 1952.
9. *Canine Medicine*, 2nd ed., Santa Barbara,

American Veterinary Publications, Inc., 1959.

10. Parry, H. B.: Structure and Development of the Retina of the Normal Dog, Brit. J. Ophthal., 37, 385, 1953.

11. Szutter, I.: *Ophthalmoskopische und Lupenspielgeluntersuchungen an Neugeborenen. Haustieren.* 1., Acta Veterinaria Academiae, Scientiarum Hungaricae, Vol. 2, Issue 2, 1961.

12. Magrane, William G.: Thesis—Canine Glaucoma, University of Pennsylvania Graduate School of Medicine, Philadelphia, 1956.

13. Troncoso, Manuel U.: *Gonioscopy*, Philadelphia, F. A. Davis Co., 1948.

Chapter 3

OCULAR THERAPEUTICS

3:1 The eye is a very delicate and sensitive organ and in applying various therapeutic preparations care must be exercised to limit the strength of applications and the manner in which they are applied. Generally speaking, almost anything used on the cornea will interfere with corneal regeneration. Ointments retard more than solutions, and powders more than ointments.

3:2 Remedies employed in the treatment of diseases of the eye may be divided into: (1) constitutional, and (2) local.

3:3 *Constitutional:* Many systemic disorders present ocular manifestations (Chapter 12), and an important part of the treatment of the latter consists in general medication intended to correct the constitutional disturbance. Several good examples of this in canine practice are: distemper, heavy internal parasite infestation, and nutritional deficiencies. It is evident that, in cases of this sort unless the systemic condition is corrected, the ocular manifestation will not respond satisfactorily.

3:4 *Local Remedies:* Drugs intended for local use are dissolved in aqueous solutions or used in oily, ointment, or powder forms. In recent years a tremendous improvement in the preparation and packaging of eye preparations has been realized. Isotonic and buffered solutions now being generally used are stable, non-irritating, sterile, and possess optimum activity. Ointment base vehicles of today are far superior to those of the past. The use of methylcellulose as the vehicle for solutions and ointments is largely responsible for this improvement.

3:5 Generally speaking, for the long term effect solutions need to be instilled more frequently than ointments. Thus, ointment preparations have usually been more popular for use by veterinarians. Solutions, however, exert a quicker effect and are often to be preferred in, for example, acute ulceration. With certain exceptions (Par. 3:65), the use of powders in the eye is to be condemned.

3:6 In applying an aqueous solution to the eye, it is best to raise the upper

31

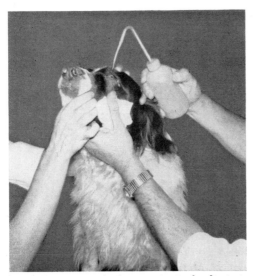

Fig. 26. Removal of secretions with plastic ir-rigating bottle.

eyedropper, undine, soft-rubber bulb syringe, or plastic irrigating bottle (Fig. 26).

3:10 Cleansing solutions recommended for home preparation and use include: (1) boric acid (1 teaspoonful in a cup of water), and (2) saline solution (1 teaspoonful NaCl in a pint of water).

3:11 An excellent cleansing, comforting solution for clinic use is:
Sodium bicarbonate ½ oz
Boric acid or Borax ½ oz
Sodium chloride ½ oz
Glycerine 2 oz
Water q.s. 1 gal. Filter or use the supernatant fluid.

3:12 To this preparation may be added 4 cc of 10 per cent Roccal or a similar quaternary ammonium chloride solution. This then becomes a 1 to 10,000 solution. Quaternary ammonium solutions of this strength are non-irritating, do not inhibit regeneration of corneal epithelium, provide a good vehicle for drugs (low surface tension), are compatible with antibiotics, and are bacteriostatic to all organisms but *E. coli* and *pyocyaneus*.

3:13 The use of plain tap water for cleansing secretions from the eye is not condoned, especially in view of the ease in which the above soothing preparation can be prepared.

lid and instill the drops just above the limbus at 12 o'clock, allowing it to flow over the cornea. If the solution is instilled into the lower cul-de-sac, it is diluted immediately with tears and passes readily into the lacrimal passages, thus a full therapeutic effect to the cornea is not obtained.

3:7 Oily solutions and ointments may be instilled into the lower cul-de-sac where they are not diluted with the tears and tend to remain longer in contact with the eye structures.

3:8 Any extended discussion of eye therapy or preparation is beyond the preview of this chapter. Only the various drugs and therapeutic measures familiar to me and proven to be of value by extensive clinical use are included.

Cleansing Solutions

3:9 Solutions of this sort are employed for flushing the conjunctival sac and removing secretions. They should be bland and used warm or at room temperature. Instillation is accomplished by

Stimulating and Astringent Remedies

3:14 These are drugs which are used locally to contract tissue and which produce a precipitate action on proteins. They are used chiefly in various forms of conjunctivitis.

3:15 Remedies in this class most frequently used are:

1. Zinc Sulfate. Its beneficial action is not so much that of an astringent but, rather, that of an irritant which restores the ability of the tissue to react to various stimuli. It is most often used in solution form and may be useful in chronic forms of conjunctivitis and in epiphora (excess tearing) of, for example, poodles.

> For clinic use and dispensing:
> Zinc sulfate 32 grains
> Boric acid 160 grains
> Distilled water q.s. 1 quart
> Sig: Several drops 2 to 3 times a day.

3:16 2. Silver Nitrate. This drug must always be dissolved in distilled water. It is most useful when used in 1 per cent solution, brushed upon the everted lids or conjunctiva in various forms of conjunctivitis. The amount to be used should be poured from the bottle to the applicator as solutions of silver nitrate spoil upon contact with organic matter.

3:17 3. Copper Sulfate. Its chief use is in the form of the crystal. This is an *especially* valuable drug for use in the chronic forms of conjunctivitis with the presence of follicles (Par. 5:42). The palpebral and bulbar conjunctiva, including both surfaces of the membrane nictitans, may be rubbed lightly with the crystal and the eye immediately flooded with the eye cleansing solution (Par. 5:36).

3:18 4. Yellow mercuric oxide is employed in an ointment (1 to 3 per cent) and is useful in blepharitis, chronic conjunctivitis, and often as an aid to the dissipation of corneal opacities associated with superficial punctate keratitis (Par. 6:37). This preparation is *never* to be used when any abrasion or ulceration of the cornea is evident.

Disinfectants and Cauterants

3:19 Disinfectants cannot be instilled into the conjunctival sac without causing injury to the cornea. They may be applied to circumscribed areas, the excess being washed off with the eye irrigating solution (Par. 3:11).

3:20 Three preparations in common use as disinfectant-cauterants are:
1. Pure carbolic acid
2. Tincture of iodine (mild to strong)
3. Trichloracetic acid (25 per cent to pure).

3:21 Disinfectant-cauterants are principally used for cauterization of corneal ulcers (Par. 6:96) or for their escharotic effect in conjunctival or corneal metaplasia (Par. 6:48).

3:22 Acids, such as carbolic, can be safely used for producing corneal sloughs because the corneal proteins are immediately precipitated by the acid.[3] This precipitate in turn acts as a barrier to the further penetration of the acid into the deeper structures of the cornea (Fig. 76). In contrast, alkalies do not form a precipitate with the proteins of the cornea, but rather pass through and in many instances cause irreparable damage.

Mydriatics and Cycloplegics

3:23 Mydriatics are agents which produce dilatation of the pupil; cycloplegics are agents which cause paralysis of the ciliary body and accommodation with a resultant dilatation of the pupil. Thus, a cycloplegic always acts as a mydriatic, but a mydriatic does not necessarily cause cycloplegia.

3:24 The most commonly used cycloplegics are atropine and homatropine. The action of homatropine is not as complete or sustained as that of atropine. The duration of action of atropine may be a week or more although pupillary effects are evident for three to five days. A noted side effect is a salivation and drooling which occurs immediately following instillation but persists for a short time only. This effect is believed to be due to irritation of the nasal mucosa.

3:25 Atropine in the sulfate form in solution or ointment form (1 to 4 per cent) is one of the most *important* and *useful* drugs in canine ophthalmology. There are few contraindications to its use, *e.g.* glaucoma, and its value in the following conditions cannot be over emphasized:

3:26 1. In iritis and uveitis, to dilate the pupil, prevent adhesions, and exert a sedative action by paralyzing the ciliary body. Ciliary spasm is an important source of pain.

3:27 2. In various diseases of the cornea, from ulceration to interstitial (deep) keratitis. Its sedative effect in these conditions is superior to that of topical anesthetics. In corneal inflammation the iris and ciliary body are usually affected to some degree. These structures share a common innervation and the ensuing iris-ciliary spasm adds to the pain and irritation of the keratopathy.

3:28 3. After certain operations, *e.g.* extracapsular cataract extraction.

3:29 4. As a mydriatic for ophthalmoscopy, although other preparations (Par. 3:30) are to be preferred because of the long lasting effect of atropine.

3:30 Mydriatics that are useful for preparing an eye for ophthalmoscopy or which may be used in an attempt to break down iritic adhesions are:

1. Tropicamide, 1.0 per cent*
2. Phenylephrine HCl, 10 per cent (viscous sol.)**
3. Cyclopentolate HCl, 1 per cent***

3:31 Tropicamide, 1 per cent has proven to be the most useful single preparation for use in canine ophthalmoscopy. Rubin's[4] investigation discloses that some of the more common preparations advocated for use in man failed to achieve the same effect in the dog.

Miotics

3:32 These drugs diminish the size of the pupil, producing tonic contraction of the sphincter of the iris and of the ciliary muscle, and reduce intraocular pressure. They are employed chiefly in glaucoma.

3:33 Preparations in common use in the past have been eserine salicylate (½ to 1 per cent) and pilocarpine hydrochloride (1 to 2 per cent) but newer preparations have proven to be vastly superior for their miotic effect in glaucoma.

3:34 Di-isopropyl fluorophosphate (D.F.P.)† 0.1 per cent in peanut oil, and Demacarium bromide 0.25 per cent‡ require fewer instillations and exert a more dramatic miotic effect (Par. 9:93, 9:94).

3:35 Eserine tends to block the action of D.F.P. and should never be used in combination. However, pilocarpine

* Mydriacyl (Alcon Laboratories, Inc., Ft. Worth, Texas).
** Neosynephrine (Winthrop Laboratories, New York, N. Y.).
*** Cyclogyl (Schieffelin and Company, New York, N. Y.).
† Floropryl (Merck Sharp & Dohme, Rahway, N. J.).
‡ Humorsol (Merck Sharp & Dohme, Rahway, N. J.).

and D.F.P. may be alternated for a more exacting miotic effect.

Local Anesthetics

3:36   Local (topical) anesthetics play an almost indispensable role in the proper examination and treatment of the eye. Preparations in common use have included cocaine, phenacaine hydrochloride (Holocaine), butacaine sulfate (Butyn), tetracaine hydrochloride (Tetracaine, Pontocaine). These drugs are effective in producing topical anesthesia, but disadvantages include severe, allergic, local reactions in the form of conjunctival chemosis (Par. 5:13) and often, a stinging sensation following instillation.

3:37   Ophthaine* has proved of real value because of its quick, efficient manner in producing topical anesthesia with complete freedom from undesirable side effects.[5]

3:38   It has been generally accepted that local anesthetics inhibit the healing process of corneal epithelium. Two preparations that do not exhibit this undesirable feature are Metycaine 2 per cent (Lilly) and Xylocaine 2 per cent (Astra),[6] and they may be used as adjunctive therapy to alleviate the pain and photophobia accompanying abrasions and ulcerations of the cornea in those cases in which atropine fails to accomplish this effect. However, there is a stinging sensation when these preparations are first instilled.

3:39   Novocaine (Procaine) 2 to 4 per cent solution is the anesthetic of choice for hypodermic use in lid growth operations or for retrobulbar injections in enucleation and intraocular surgery in conjunction with general anesthesia.

* Ophthaine (E. R. Squibb & Sons, New York, N. Y.).

Antibiotics and Chemotherapy

3:40   Antibiotics and the sulfanamides have an important place in the treatment and prevention of ocular infections.[7] In order to achieve optimum results, however, one must know: (1) the penetrating properties into the eye and through the blood aqueous barrier, (2) the sensitivities and resistance, and (3) the spectrum they encompass. Studies as regards toxicities or effectiveness elsewhere in the body mean little, *e.g.* penicillin may be effective in a streptococcic infection of the throat, but that same organism in the eye will not be affected by penicillin since this particular antibiotic penetrates the blood aqueous barrier of the eye very poorly.

3:41   An appreciation of the importance and a knowledge of the function of the blood aqueous barrier of the eye is essential. This barrier differs from the blood tissue barriers in the rest of the body, except for perhaps the brain, because of the low concentration of protein in the aqueous as opposed to its much higher concentration in all other tissues.

3:42   In diseases of the eye, then, there are additional problems because of the peculiarities of the blood aqueous barrier. The presence of adequate blood concentrations in the body does not guarantee adequate concentrations in all ocular fluids and tissues that may be involved in the infectious process. In other words, we must be concerned not only with whether or not the organism responsible for the infection in the ocular tissue is susceptible to the drug chosen, but whether the drug will penetrate into the involved ocular tissues in sufficient concentration to bring about the desired result.

3:43   Most of the commonly used

antibiotics, *e.g.* penicillin, streptomycin, aureomycin, and terramycin, must be given in massive doses and by injection to feebly penetrate the blood aqueous barrier. Neither do they penetrate an intact corneal epithelium. They do, however, penetrate an abraded epithelium.

3:44   Chloramphenicol, on the other hand, is absorbed rapidly, secreted slowly and penetrates the blood aqueous barrier readily when given orally.[8] It also penetrates an intact epithelium when applied locally.

3:45   Neomycin, bacitracin, and polymyxin, in addition to the aforementioned antibiotics, are all used topically to treat infections with sensitive organisms. However, if the infection is severe or intraocular in nature, systemic treatment with chloramphenicol is imperative.

3:46   Sulfonamides have largely been supplanted by the antibiotics, but they are still very useful and more of their mode of action is understood. In the local use of sulfonamides, these points must be kept in mind.

3:47   (1) Their efficacy is impeded by the presence of pus and other secretions containing large amounts of para-aminobenzoic acid, and irrigation of the conjunctival sac should be employed before instillation. High concentrations should be used, *e.g.* sulfacetamide sodium (30 per cent).

3:48   (2) Regeneration of corneal epithelium is retarded by sulfonamides, and for this reason it is not wise to use these drugs after extensive corneal abrasions, or at least for only a limited time.

3:49   Sodium sulfacetamide appears to possess the best power of penetrating the intact corneal epithelium, but when the cornea is infected, its permeability is altered and all sulfonamides pass through readily. When used systemically, the sulfonamides penetrate the blood aqueous barrier and diffuse readily into all ocular tissue.

Steroids

3:50   Perhaps the greatest usefulness of the corticosteroids in veterinary medicine lies in the field of ophthalmology.[9] This importance has become manifest primarily because good therapeutic results depend upon sufficient amounts of the steroids reaching the sites where needed. Since the eye is readily accessible, optimum results can be expected.

3:51   However, enthusiasm must be tempered with the realization that there are definite contraindications to their use.[10] Steroids do not affect the causative agents but rather the tissue response to those agents. They *do not* have antibiotic or chemotherapeutic effect, but, even when combined with a suitable antibiotic, there still are contraindications to their use, *e.g.* acute ulceration (Par. 6:102).

3:52   The ocular effects of steroid therapy are to:
1. Suppress hypersensitivity reactions
2. Suppress ocular reactions to irritants
3. Suppress inflammatory processes as result of infections
4. Suppress neovascularization of the cornea
5. Reduce fibroblastic activity in the cornea
6. Interfere with effective immunological reactions.

Uses

3:53   It is important to delineate the specific fields of action.[11] The topical preparations (drops and ointments) are not absorbed in sufficient strength to benefit intraocular conditions. Thus their use is limited to the anterior segment (external ocular inflammations and allergies).

3:54 Topical instillation and/or subconjunctival injections:
(1) lid and conjunctival allergies and diseases
(2) superficial keratitis (vascularization, pannus, exuberant granulation tissue
(3) episcleritis
(4) postoperative.

3:55 Systemic and/or subconjunctival injection:
(1) Interstitial (deep) keratitis
(2) Iritis
(3) Amaurosis.

3:56 Methods of administration (Prednisolone preparations)
1. Drops (topical suspension) 0.25 per cent up. Instilled as often as every two hours.
2. Ointments—0.5 per cent (5 mg/gm) up to 1.5 per cent (15 mg/gm). Instilled every eight hours.
3. Subconjunctival injection—2.5 to 5 mg injection is made at forty-eight-hour intervals. Technique: Adequate topical anesthesia is first obtained. Then, using a 25 gauge needle (¼ to ½ in) mounted on a 1 cc hypo, the injection is made underneath the bulbar conjunctiva at any accessible area (Fig. 27). The needle is twisted on withdrawal to prevent leakage. A bleb results which usually subsides within a few hours. The repeat injections are given at different sites.
4. Systemic. This administration may be either by intramuscular injection or per orum. Dosage depends upon the preparation used.

Vitamins

3:57 In ophthalmology we are concerned with vitamin therapy, especially in those avitaminoses due to the absence or insufficient amount of vitamins A, C, and riboflavin and niacin of the B complex.

3:58 Vitamin A assumes an extremely important role in the physiology of vision.[12] In vitamin A deficiency, various tissues all over the body begin to deteriorate, the retina included. The rods in the retinal fundus exhibit

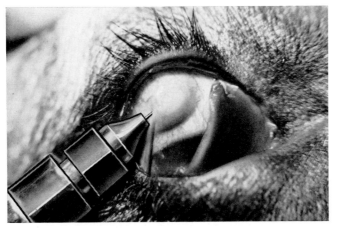

Fig. 27. Bleb arising from a subconjunctival injection.

marked changes and, as the deficiency progresses, other layers of the retina become involved. Fortunately, however, even rods which have degenerated completely appear to regenerate within two to four months of vitamin A administration.

3:59   Vitamin A is also thought necessary and essential for the normal life of the epithelial cell. In the absence of this vitamin, these cells degenerate and atrophy, followed by a proliferation on the part of the basal cells, resulting in keratinization and keratomalacia (Par. 6:92).

3:60   Vitamin C (ascorbic acid) is essential for the proper maintenance of intercellular cement substances. In vitamin C deficiency the characteristic lesion is the occurrence of capillary hemorrhages due to the failure of the endothelial cells to produce cement substance and thus allowing the capillaries to rupture. This vitamin is also important to the regeneration of corneal epithelium and is useful in ulcerative keratitis.

3:61   Riboflavin (B$_2$) deficiency is characterized by superficial vascularization with a possible ulceration and subsequent opacity of the cornea.

3:62   Niacin is believed to enhance the regeneration of corneal epithelium and, thus, is also useful in the therapy of ulcerative keratitis.

3:63   *Dosage*
Vitamin A   25,000 to 50,000 units daily
Vitamin C   50 to 150 mg daily
Riboflavin   5 to 15 mg daily
Niacin   50 to 150 mg daily

3:64   Daily administration of a therapeutic capsule containing approximate amounts of the above vitamins constitutes good adjunctive therapy in cases of corneal ulceration or ocular manifestations resulting from improper nutrition or debilitating disease.

Other Therapeutic Measures

3:65   Dionin, a derivative of morphine, is an analgesic used in iritis, glaucoma, and keratitis. It relieves deep-seated pain acting as a vasodilator. It has occasionally been used as an aid to the absorption of corneal opacities when steroids have failed to do so. Since it produces a marked chemosis and swelling of the lids when first instilled, a 2 per cent solution is first prescribed, followed in a day or so by a 10 per cent solution, and, finally, by application of a few grains of the powder to the cornea.

3:66   *Carbonic anhydrase inhibitors*° have proven to be a most useful addition to the treatment of glaucoma as they lower intraocular pressure by inhibiting secretion of the aqueous (Par. 9:90). They are also useful, because of this feature, when given prior to the performance of intraocular surgery.

3:67   *Enzymes.* Chymar (Armour) has been useful as an intramuscular injection for aid in the absorption of intraocular debris (hypopyon, hyphema).

3:68   *Fluorescein* is used to detect abrasions, infiltrations, and ulceration of the cornea and to define the limits of such lesions. The methods of use include a 2 per cent aqueous solution or sterile impregnated papers. The latter method (Fig. 17, Chapter 2) is preferred as the solution is a good culture media for *Pseudomonas* and has been known to inoculate eyes with disastrous results.[13, 14]

° Cardrase (Upjohn). Daranide (Merck Sharp & Dohme). Diamox (Lederle).

3:69 *Non-Specific Protein Therapy.* Milk and typhoid-paratyphoid vaccine are the foreign proteins that are routinely used in ophthalmology. Foreign proteins supposedly stimulate or increase the antibodies thus increasing the natural resistance against the invading bacteria. It should only be used as adjunct therapy. Preparations that have on occasion proved to be useful include: (1) Sterile milk, 5 cc i.m. repeated every two to three days, increasing the amount as indicated. (2) Omnadin (Conc.-Winthrop) 2 cc as above. (3) Typhoid vaccine (i.v.) 15,000,000 organisms at the first dose, rest a day, 30,000,000 organisms, rest a day, then 60,000,000 organisms.

3:70 The indications for foreign protein therapy are: infected corneal ulcers, severe iritis and uveitis and some cases of purulent conjunctivitis.

3:71 *Heat.* Hot, moist compresses are prescribed in affections of the cornea, iris, ciliary body, sclera and orbit as a whole. Hot cloths are usually applied on the closed lids and renewed every few minutes for 15 minutes several times a day. Heat is a vasodilator producing an active hyperemia with an increase of leukocytes and antibodies and thus aiding in the absorption of inflammatory products.

3:72 *Cold.* Moist, cold compresses are of distinct benefit to those injuries of the eyelids, eyes and surrounding tissues that produce swelling and pain and are sometimes accompanied by hemorrhage. As a vasoconstrictor it produces an ischemia in tissues that are swollen, chemotic or edematous, thereby hastening recovery.

3:73 *Electrocautery* (Fig. 28). I have become most enthusiastic with the use of electrocautery and coagulation for: (1) removal of distorted or unwanted cilia causing distichiasis, trichiasis (Par. 4:33), (2) mild entropion (Par. 4:21), (3) removal of lid tumors (Par. 4:75), (4) peritomy (Par. 6:51), and (5) cautery in intraocular surgical procedures, including iridectomy (Par. 7:81).

3:74 *Radiation.* X-ray or beta ray therapy has been well investigated and utilized in canine ophthalmology.[15–17] Although radiation still is useful adjunct therapy, its importance has been lessened with the development and use of the newer steroid preparations.

3:75 Regardless of whether x-ray or beta ray is used for therapy, the tissue effects are identical. Beta ray (Fig. 29), however, offers important advantages over x-ray, namely, (1) ease of administration, (2) greater safety for both operator and patient, and (3) heavier dosages in much less time and with little danger of consequent postradiation cataract formation.

3:76 Conditions which respond to radiation of either type are (1) early pannus, with or without accompanying pigmentation, (2) neovascularization of the cornea, irrespective of cause, (3) exuberant granulation of the cornea, (4) pre- and postoperatively in keratectomy procedures, and (5) small neoplasms of lids, conjunctiva or cornea.

3:77 Definite contraindications include (1) acute ulcer formation and (2) the direct application of the beta applicator to any ulcerative process.

3:78 The limbus is the preferable site (Fig. 30) for administering the beta rays. Scattered x-radiation to the globe as a whole is the rule. Smaller doses and repeated applications of the beta rays are preferred to single, large doses.

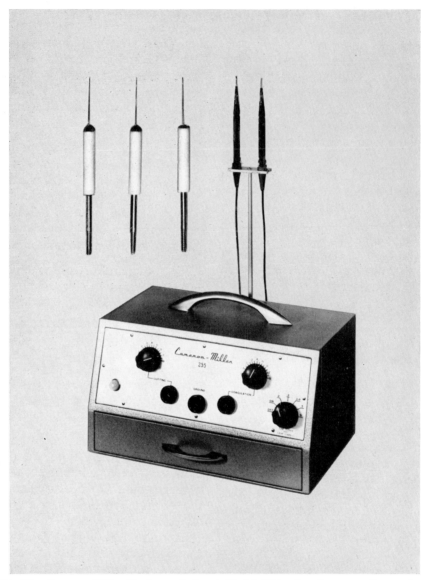

Fig. 28. The Cameron-Miller Electrosurgical unit Model 255 and epilation needles used in distichiasis and trichiasis.

Total massive dosages (50,000 R.E.P. or over), even when divided into interval doses, appear to be no more efficacious than small, divided administrations.

3:79 X-ray dosages should not exceed 600 r total with single doses of from 100 to 150 at three- or four-day intervals being employed most commonly.

3:80   *Bandaging.* With an ordinary amount of patience and practice, the eye or eyes of most breeds can be easily bandaged. A comfortable bandage will be well tolerated and offers three important advantages: (1) immobilization of the globe, (2) extra warmth (conducive to healing), and (3) prevention of infection.

3:81 A sterile piece of combined roll or fracture padding can be held in place by an elastic type adhesive* or stockinette (Fig. 31). Eyes are routinely bandaged following intraocular surgery and, when possible, following iris prolapse surgery. Bandaging is also useful following a keratectomy or non-healing abrasions and ulcerations.

3:82 *Fungicides.* Diseases in which the fungi have assumed an important role are on the increase. The one clinical denominator in these recent cases has been the use of antibiotics and steroids. Antibiotics enhance fungus growth by inhibition of the normal bacterial flora, while steroids facilitate fungus proliferation through interference with the host's anti-inflammatory and immune responses.

3:83 Thus, dogs afflicted with chronic keratopathies in which antibiotic steroid combinations have been used over a long period often develop a conjunctival discharge which, when

* Elasticon (Johnson and Johnson).

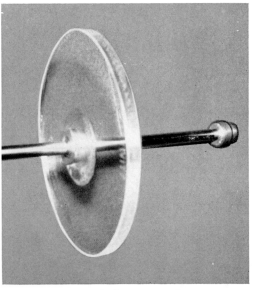

Fig. 29. The beta-ray applicator.

cultured, reveal fungus growth. In these instances switching to preparations such as Panolog (Squibb) which contain fungicides in addition to the steroid-antibiotic, will alleviate the condition.

3:84 Sodium Proprionate** has also

** Proprian (Wyeth).

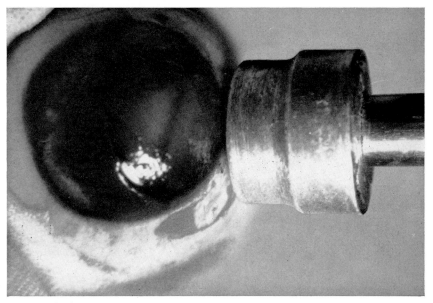

Fig. 30. The beta-ray source in position at the limbus following a superficial keratectomy.

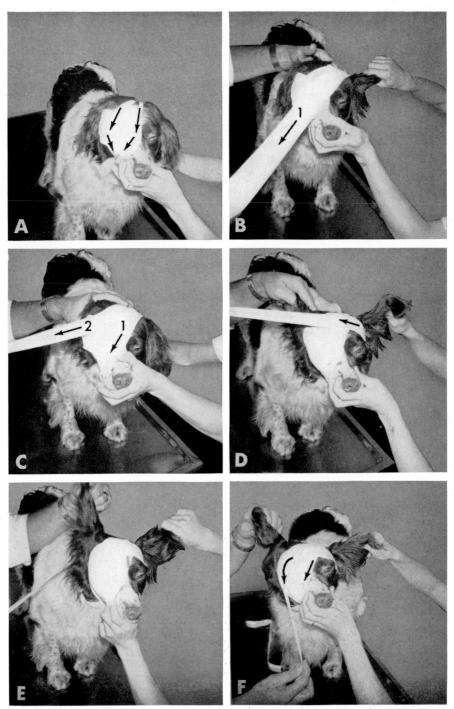

Fig. 31. Method of bandaging with pad and elastic adhesive. *A.* The pad is held in place by a continuous strip of adhesive, starting at the base of the opposite ear, to include the medial and lateral aspects of the pad. *B.* Depending upon head size, 1 or 2 inch Elasticon is started at the base of the opposite ear. The assistant retains hold on a corner of the eye pad at all times. The first roll of the bandage (1) should just miss the commissure of the mouth. *C.* A second roll (2) around the head is made to encompass the lateral aspect of the pad. Then the roll is brought under the jaw to and around the temple in front of the ear on the opposite side. *D.* The roll is continued to the opposite temple and in front of the ear on the bandaged side. *E.* The roll is then continued around the neck back of the ears. This roll, then, is parallel with the support encircling the head in front of the ears. *F.* A final strip of adhesive is used to "nail down" the medial aspect of the bandage. Inclusion of some hair along this border helps to prevent slippage. The strip is continued around the lateral aspect of the bandage.

42

been useful as a bacteriostatic and fungistatic eyewash.

3:85 *Antihistamines.* Useful in allergic conditions of the lids and conjunctiva but their popularity has lessened with the increased use of the steroids. Steroid-antihistamine preparations are available under many trade names.

3:86 *Castor Oil and Cod Liver Oil* are soothing preparations which can be recommended for first aid use. They are useful for protection prior to bathing, can be used following minor abrasions of the cornea and conjunctiva, and following cauterization of ulcers.

3:87 *Anticoagulants.* Heparin (1 minim) is occasionally instilled in the anterior chamber to discourage clot and fibrin formation following intraocular surgery. Its use may predispose to additional hemorrhage, however.

3:88 *Coagulants.* Systemic preparations which have proven of value in decreasing capillary permeability are C.V.P. with K* and Adrenosem.** This type therapy is indicated in certain cases of hyphema (Par. 11:12).

3:89 *Adrenalin.* The vasoconstrictor

* U. S. Vitamin Corp.
** Massengill.

action is useful in the control of hemorrhages both from the smaller arterioles and the capillaries of the conjunctiva, and for the relief of congested mucous membranes. When injected subconjunctivally, it may release recent iritic adhesions and dilate the pupil. Adrenalin in the 1 to 1,000 solution is most useful throughout intraocular surgical procedures and for instillation into the anterior chamber to encourage dilation following extracapsular cataract extraction (Par. 10:94).

3:90 *Artificial Tears.* Methylcellulose*** is commonly used in from 0.5 to 1 per cent solution as artificial tears and as a soothing base for many ophthalmic preparations. It has a minimum effect on regeneration of corneal epithelium and has the important feature of increasing corneal contact time by a considerable margin over non-methylcellulose solutions.

3:91 Artificial tears can be purchased under several different trade names. The bulk powder may also be purchased and a stock solution made for use as artificial tears or as a vehicle for numerous ophthalmic preparations the clinician may want to prepare.

*** Methocel 4000 CPS USP (Dow Chemical Co.).

GENERAL CONSIDERATIONS FOR EYE SURGERY

3:92 Ocular surgery can be divided into two parts: extraocular and intraocular. Essentially, extraocular surgery involves procedures of the lids, conjunctiva and cornea which are easily performed by the veterinarian possessing the qualifications essential to general surgery. Intraocular surgery (*e.g.* cataract, glaucoma procedures), on the other hand, demands the skills of a person willing to devote an unusual

amount of time to the study of a specific specialty.

3:93 The intraocular surgeon must be temperamentally suited and have patience. It is not sufficient to simply be an accomplished surgeon. To achieve any degree of success he must be well versed in medical ophthalmology, and have an intimate knowledge and a thorough understanding of the surgical

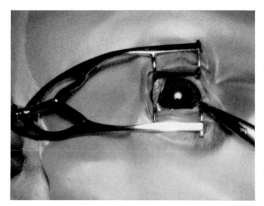

Fig. 32. The use of rubber dental dam and the eye speculum for draping.

anatomy of the eye. A distance of 1 mm may not be critical in performing an incision elsewhere in the body, but it can mean the difference between success or failure in an eye operation. In addition, a knowledge of ophthalmic pathology is a most important aid in the proper selection of cases. For example, some cataract extractions, even though properly executed, are doomed to failure without this knowledge (Par. 10:33).

3:94   Other considerations which are important to the degree of success are: adequate practice surgery, a sufficient number of cases for perfection of a technique, and religiously adhering to the time-proven procedures of preoperative care, surgical techniques, and postoperative care practiced by ophthalmologists in human medicine.

3:95   The rules of asepsis and antisepsis which govern general surgery are also indicated in ophthalmic operations. This is especially true in consideration of intraocular procedures where introduction of infection, a cilia, lint, glove powder, etc., will nullify the best effort. By following a very rigid aseptic routine and utilizing the aid of a well-trained assistant, many complications leading to failure can be avoided.

3:96   It is most important that the area about the eye is prepared properly and that the eye is draped in such a manner that skin and lid exposure is minimized. A small sheet of rubber dental dam with a slit cut for insertion of the eye speculum is included in the pack for this purpose, and is used to envelop the lids and skin area left exposed by the head and body drape (Fig. 32).

Preparation of the Patient

3:98   In a preoperative evaluation and preparation, any discharge other than normal tearing should be noted by the surgeon. Intraocular surgery should not be performed in the presence of infection. The actual preparation of the patient is begun at least twenty-four hours prior to surgery:

1. Instill an antibiotic ointment in the lower cul-de-sac, allowing a film of the ointment to form over the cornea. This film is for protective purposes prior to steps 2, 3, and 4.

2. Clip the hair with surgical blade approximately 1½ to 2 inches back from the upper and lower lids, as well as the lateral commissure of the lids. Brush or vacuum loose hair away.

3. With blunt point scissors, the blades of which have been anointed with either water or mineral oil, cut the lashes of the upper lid. Lashes will cling to the scissors.

4. With a cotton ball, rub straight surgical soap into the clipped areas around the lids. Wet a ball of cotton, squeeze out excess water, work up a lather, and with succeeding balls of wet cotton remove all evidences of dirt and soap.

5. Irrigate eye and lids of any remaining hair or lashes.

6. Dry lids with cotton, apply alcohol, and instill into the cul-de-sac the previously used antibiotic ophthalmic oint-

ment, also massaging same into the clipped area around the eye.

7. If surgery is for cataract extraction, use atropine solution or ointment prior to step 6.

8. Several times before surgery the ointment application and atropine (if cataract) is repeated as in step 6.

Ordinarily the administration of a carbonic anhydrase inhibitor to lower intraocular tension (Par. 3:66) is included in the preoperative preparation, the final dose being given several hours before surgery.

Positioning of the Patient

3:99 Position depends somewhat on the procedure to be performed. Basically, however, the dog is placed on its side with the eye to be operated uppermost. The head should be at the end of the table and supported in the desired position by sand bags or rolled newspaper (Fig. 33). Elevation of the nose is often sufficient. With the head at the end of the table, the instrument stand is within easy reach of the surgeon and assistant (Fig. 34).

The Operating Room

3:100 The design of an ophthalmic operating room need not be different from that of a general surgery but the lighting requirements are different. Intraocular surgery cannot be satisfactorily performed in a brilliantly lighted room since this type of light tends to produce a reflection from the cornea, making it impossible to see details within the anterior chamber. Artificial focal illumination in a darkened room is essential.

Instruments

3:101 The instruments used in eye surgery are similar to those used in general surgery, but are much smaller to allow for greater precision in their manipulation.

3:102 Most eye surgical instruments are very delicate and utmost care must be exercised in their handling and sterilization. The cutting edges, grasping teeth and other functional parts must not strike other objects. Sterilization can be accomplished in the usual way, but dry heat has proven to be the best, especially as regards preservation of cutting edges. After use, instruments should be thoroughly cleaned as soon as practical, removing all residue with hot water, soap or a non-corrosive solvent. Cleaning of sharp instruments and for-

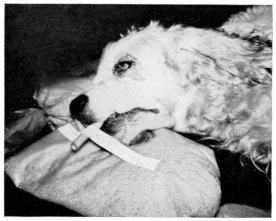

Fig. 33. The head positioned for eye surgery using plastic bags filled with "kitty litter."

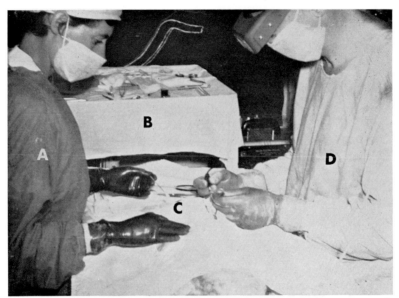

Fig. 34.   Positions assumed for surgery on the left eye. *A*. Assistant. *B*. Instrument stand accessible to assistant and surgeon.

C. Dog's head under the drape. *D*. Surgeon sitting and with forearms steaded on drape-covered sand bags.

ceps with delicate teeth should be done with as little wiping as possible. Storage in cases is recommended, especially when infrequent use is anticipated.

3:103   Ophthalmic instruments are many and varied but a good basic set (Fig. 35) includes: Castroviejo eye speculum (medium), straight blunt strabismus or tenotomy scissors, dull iris hook, 2 rat tooth curved mosquito forceps, several lacrimal cannulas, Mc-Guire corneal scissors, Graefe strabismus hook (medium), eye dressing forceps (straight serrated), tissue forceps (1 and 2 teeth), fixation forceps with catch, eye needle holder, Beaver blades #64 and 65 and handles* (Fig. 36). Finally, suitable magnification (Fig. 9, Chapter 2) must be used by the surgeon. It is impossible to work within millimeters without this aid.

3:104   In addition to the instruments required for a specific operation a pack usually also includes:

* Beaver, 480 Trapelo Rd., Belmont 79, Mass.

cotton applicators
irrigation jar and bulbs
5–0 chromic catgut
eye pad
2 and 5 cc hypodermic syringes with
    25 and 20 gauge needles
needles and suture material for the
    lids
rubber dam

3:105   6–0 silk or mersilene* are used for closure in intraocular procedures. Greishaber (#81) 7 mm needles are the sharpest obtainable and ideally suited for use in the tough corneal-scleral structures of the dog. Atraumatic 6–0 silk sutures and needles are satisfactory for use in certain procedures where the structures are weakened and thinned by age or absolute glaucoma.

Anesthesia

3:106   Ordinarily, general anesthesia is to be preferred in most extraocular procedures and when performing any

** Ethicon (Code R-51), Somerville, N. J.

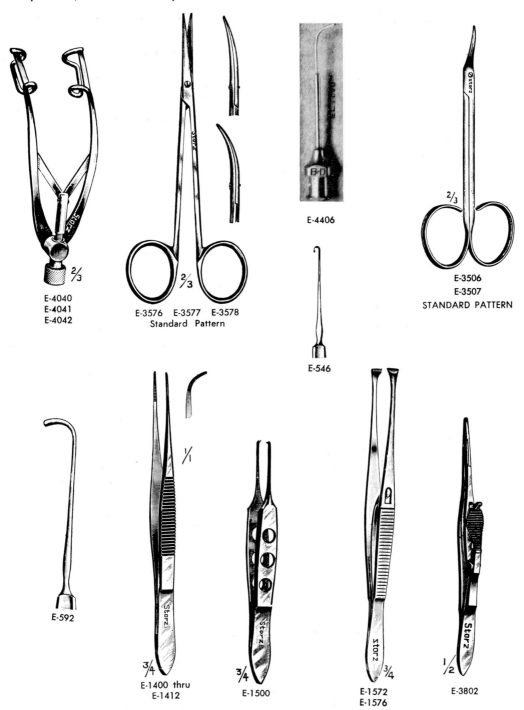

E-4040
E-4041
E-4042

E-3576   E-3577   E-3578
Standard Pattern

E-4406

E-546

E-3506
E-3507
STANDARD PATTERN

E-592

E-1400 thru
E-1412

E-1500

E-1572
E-1576

E-3802

Fig. 35.   Basic set of instruments.

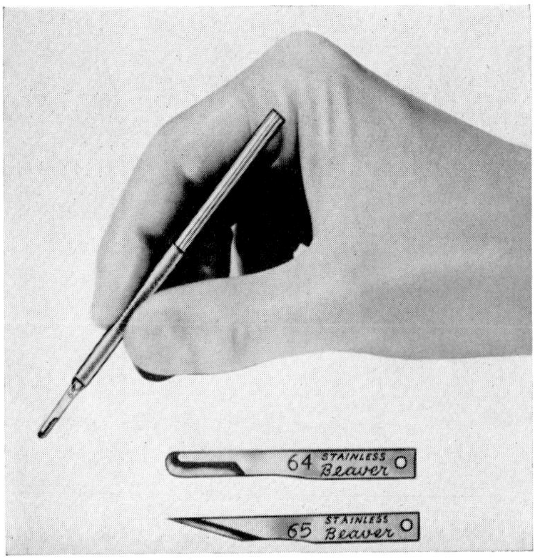

Fig. 36.   Beaver mini-blades and handle.

an antibiotic. Dressings are usually changed daily so that the eye can be further medicated.

References

1. Allen, James H.: *May's Diseases of the Eye*, 23rd ed., Baltimore, The Williams & Wilkins Co., 1963.
2. Harrison, William J.: *Ocular Therapeutics*, 2nd ed., Springfield, Charles C Thomas, 1953.
3. Magrane, William G.: Ocular Physiology—Clinical Application, No. Am. Vet., *36*, p. 389, 1955.
4. Rubin, Lionel F. and Wolfes, Robert L.: Mydriatics for Canine Ophthalmoscopy, J.A.V.M.A., *140*, p. 137, 1962.
5. Magrane, William G.: Investigational Use of Ophthaine as a Local Anesthetic in Ophthalmology, No. Am. Vet., *34*, p. 568, 1953.
6. Marr, W. G. *et al.*: Effect of Topical Anesthetics on Regeneration of Corneal Epithelium, Am. J. Ophthal., *43*, p. 606, 1957.
7. Magrane, William G.: An Evaluation of the Use of Antibiotics in Canine Ophthalmology, No. Am. Vet., *32*, p. 169, 1951.
8. Magrane, William G.: The Clinical Use of Chloromycetin in Canine Ocular Infections, No. Am. Vet., *34*, p. 39, 1953.
9. Magrane, William G.: Cortisone in Ophthalmology, No. Am. Vet., *32*, p. 763, 1951.
10. Magrane, William G.: The Use of Corticoids in Ophthalmology, Abstracts of First Veterinary Symposium on the Use of Meticorten and Meticortelone, Schering Corp., Bloomfield, New Jersey, 1956.
11. Gordon, Dan M.: *The Clinical Use of Corticotropin, Cortisone and Hydrocortisone in Eye Disease*, Springfield, Charles C Thomas, 1954.
12. Wald, G.: The Photoreceptor Process in Vision, Am. J. Ophthal., *40*, p. 36, 1955.
13. Cello, Robert M. and Lasmanis, J.: Pseudomonas Infection of the Eye of the Dog Resulting from the Use of Contaminated Fluorescein Solution, J.A.V.M.A., *132*, p. 297, 1958.
14. Kirmura, S. J.: Fluorescein Paper, Am. J. Ophthal., *34*, p. 466, 1957.
15. Magrane, William G.: X-ray Therapy in Interstitial and Pigmentary Keratitis, No. Am. Vet., *29*, p. 582, 1948.
16. Magrane, William G.: Beta ray and x-ray Therapy in Diseases of the Eye, No. Am. Vet., *36*, p. 295, 1955.
17. Michaelson, S.: The Use of Beta Irradiation in Veterinary Ophthalmology, Vet. Med., *49*, p. 475, 1954.

intraocular operation. The type of general anesthesia used is, of course, dependent upon the procedure and the individual preference of the surgeon. I have found the following routine to be most satisfactory.

1. Pre-anesthetic sedation with morphine-atropine one hour before.

2. Intravenous pentobarbital, short acting barbiturate or a combination of the two, depending on age of patient and length of the procedure.

3. Ringers-dextrose tubing is attached to the i.v. needle. This slow drip offers the usual advantages, including ready access for administration of any further anesthetic required.

4. Intubation tube inserted and left in until the patient starts to arouse.

5. An intramuscular injection of a tranquilizer is given at or shortly following the completion of surgery to insure an excitement-free recovery.

3:107   *Bandaging* (Par. 3:81), when indicated, is performed immediately following surgery and the instillation of

Chapter 4

DISEASES AND SURGERY OF THE LIDS AND LACRIMAL APPARATUS

Anatomy and Physiology

4:1   The eyelids consist of movable folds of skin, loose connective tissue, muscular tissue, tarsus, and conjunctiva (Fig. 37). These dorsal and ventral folds form the *palpebral fissure*. The lids present protective eyelashes (cilia) at their margins, and contain numerous glands, blood vessels, lymphatics and nerves. They serve the purpose of excluding light from the eyes, sweep away foreign bodies reaching the cornea, spread lacrimal fluid and lubricant from their accessory glands over the cornea (*precorneal film*) and aid in the drainage of this fluid through the drainage channels by a pumping action. The

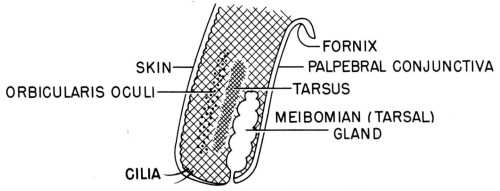

Fig. 37.   Longitudinal section of the upper lid.

49

upper eyelid is more movable than the lower.

4:2   The eyelids form a medial and lateral canthi. Opposite the medial canthus lies a tuft of long tactile hairs. Near this medial commissure (4 to 6 mm) are the two *puncta lacrimalia* (Fig. 38) through which the lacrimal fluid drains into the connecting *canaliculi,* thence to the *lacrimal sac* and *nasolacrimal duct* (Fig. 39). This structure is known as the *excretory* portion of the lacrimal apparatus. The puncta are, in reality, slit-like openings set well back from the lid margins and turned in slightly towards the eye. The two openings are not always the same size and it is not uncommon for one or both to be absent (Par. 4:50). The lacrimal sac lies in the lacrimal fossa of the medial orbital wall. The sac is not as well developed in the dog as it is in man. From the sac area the fluid flows along the nasolacrimal duct within the nasolacrimal canal into the nasal cavity.

4:3   The *secretory* portion of the lacrimal apparatus includes the *lacrimal gland* (tear production) and the microscopic accessory glands (precorneal film production). The lacrimal gland is located in the supra-orbital fossa on the dorsolateral aspect of the eyeball (Par. 8:10) (Fig. 39). Excretory ducts empty their contents into the conjunctival sac upon sympathetic stimulation.

4:4   The fluid normally found in the conjunctival cul-de-sac is, then, a mixture of the secretions of the lacrimal gland and accessory lacrimal glands. Any physicochemical change in the component parts of these secretions influences the health of the underlying corneal stroma. The precorneal film secretion is viscid, high in protein, with a low surface tension, and is very important to the well-being of the cornea (Par. 6:55). Tears, too, are high in protein and have a low surface tension, which enables them to wet the epithelial surfaces thoroughly. Aside from

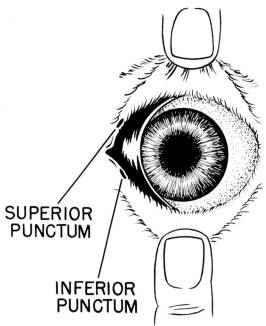

SUPERIOR PUNCTUM

INFERIOR PUNCTUM

Fig. 38.   The puncta lacrimalia.

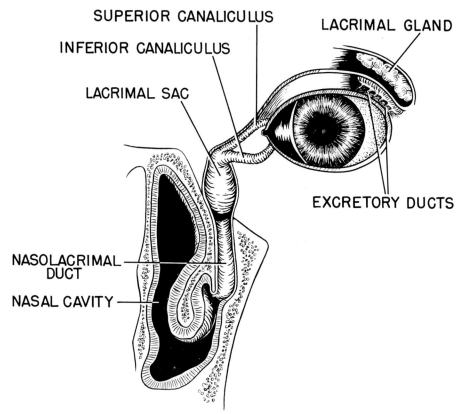

Fig. 39.   The lacrimal production and drainage system.

the lubricating qualities, however, tears in themselves are bactericidal and contain lysozyme, an enzyme that dissolves many airborne saprophytes rapidly and completely.[1]

4:5   The underlying structures of the eyelids include the well-developed *orbicularis muscle* which is found almost to the edge of each eyelid, and always nearest the anterior surface, thickening at the root of the eyelid.

4:6   Posterior to the orbicularis muscle is a layer of dense connective tissue called the *tarsus*. The tarsal plate serves to give the eyelids rigidity but is not as well developed in the dog as it is in man. In close opposition to the tarsus is a series of glands (tarsal or meibomian).

4:7   The *meibomian glands*[2] are plainly visible through the conjunctiva as pale parallel lines running vertically to the upper edge of the tarsal plate from the lid margins. Their outlets can be seen as tiny apertures along the inner lid margins. Their secretion is more viscous than lacrimal fluid, and functions as a dam against the overflow of the latter before it reaches the puncta.

4:8   Finally, the inner surface of the eyelid is covered by mucous membrane, the *palpebral* conjunctiva.

Congenital Anomalies

4:9   *Coloboma* of the lid is a notching of the margin with an absence of the lashes and glands in the affected

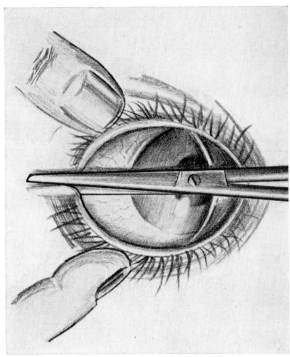

Fig. 40.   Canthotomy.

area. It is rarely encountered and can be treated, if necessary, by plastic methods. *Dermoid cyst,* a congenital tumor, occupies space at what would normally be the lateral canthus aspect of the lid commissure. This condition is more fully discussed in Paragraph 4:75.

4:10   *Narrow Palpebral Fissure.* This particular anomaly is not uncommon in terriers, *e.g.* Kerry Blue terriers, and Chows, and is often responsible for the development of a subsequent entropion. Enlargement of the palpebral fissure by canthotomy and canthoplasty will often suffice to correct the entropion without an additional entropion procedure.

4:11   *Canthotomy* is the temporary enlargement of the palpebral fissure by severing the lateral canthus and is used as a preliminary measure to other surgical procedures. A narrow palpebral fissure may be enlarged prior to or during intraocular or orbital operations.[3]

4:12   The technique is simple and consists of stretching the lateral canthus between the thumb and forefinger and cutting the canthus for the desired distance with heavy blunt-pointed scissors (Fig. 40). Hemorrhage attending the procedure can be minimized by first injecting a few minims of 1 to 1,000 epinephrine at the canthus or crushing the canthus for thirty seconds or so with a hemostatic forceps.

4:13   When only a canthotomy is performed, *i.e.* as an adjunct to intraocular or orbital operations, the incision may be left to heal of its own accord or is sutured if more rapid healing is desired.

4:14   *Canthoplasty* results in a permanent lengthening of the palpebral fissure. Smythe[4] describes a technique that, with modification, has worked well for me. Following the canthotomy procedure, a portion of skin above, below, and opposite the commissure is removed (Fig. 41A). The upper and lower lateral lid margins are then separated from their underlying structures for the required distance and the skin is undermined in the immediate area (Fig. 41B). The upper and lower lid edges are then sutured separately to the intact skin margin, forming the new lateral commissure. Several supporting dorsal and ventral sutures complete the repair (Fig. 41C). 5–0 Dermalon attached to atraumatic needles has proven a suitable suture for plastic lid surgery.

4:15   This technique not only provides a wider palpebral fissure, but offers a good cosmetic result in that the lid margins have been extended to the commissure. Other procedures for elongating the palpebral fissure are described fully in the many texts of human ophthalmic surgery.

4:16   *Large Palpebral Fissure.* Too large an opening may enclose a normal eye, *e.g.* in English bulldogs, spaniels,

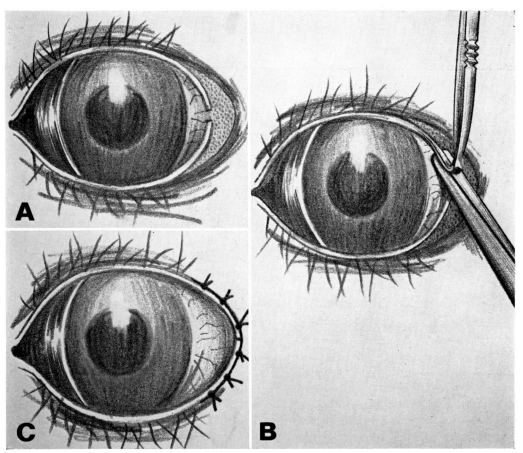

Fig. 41.   Canthoplasty. *A.* Skin is removed above, below, and opposite the lateral canthus.
B. Lid margins are loosened. *C.* Lid margins sutured to the skin, forming a new lateral canthus.

hounds, resulting in an ectropic condition.

Congenital or Acquired Conditions

Entropion (Plate 2A)

4:17   *Entropion* is simply defined as an inrolling of the lid (and with it the lashes). *Etiology.* It may be an acquired condition as a result of cicatricial contraction following injuries or a chronic conjunctivitis with blepharospasm, but in the dog it most often is seen as a congenital anomaly in Chows and the hunting breeds. Usually only the lower lid is involved, but it occasionally becomes necessary to affect correction of both upper and lower lids by one of several means.

4:18   *Symptoms.* Entropion results in superficial irritation of the bulbar conjunctiva and cornea producing a chronic discharge, vascularization and possible ulceration of the cornea. Neglect and/or rubbing by the animal can lead to erosion of the corneal stroma, prolapse of the iris and loss of an eye. Painful frequent blinking and photophobia characterize the subjective symptoms.

4:19   *Treatment: Medical.* A mild acquired entropion associated with a disease process may respond to subconjunctival steroid injections with follow-up of topical steroid-antibiotic combinations. Mineral oil injections into the lid have been used in attempts to correct entropion. This procedure is not to be recommended because of the likelihood of producing foreign body granuloma at the site of the injection.[5]

4:20   *Surgery.* Many operative procedures with multiple variations have been advocated for the correction of entropion. The following embrace the principles of correction and are those with which the author is most familiar.

4:21   1. *Cautery-puncture.* Cautery-puncture is effective only in entropion of limited degree and may need to be repeated. It is often of value when only a portion of the lid is involved. A tongue depressor or suitable substitute is placed behind the lid to protect the underlying eyeball. The skin of the lower lid is penetrated with a blunt pointed electrode or well-heated strabismus (muscle) hook. These punctures, in one or two rows, are 4 to 5 mm from the lid margin and extend into the tarsal area of the lid but not through the palpebral conjunctiva (Fig. 42). The resultant cicatrization results in eversion.

4:22   2. *Skin Excision.* (1) Trephine removal of skin plugs utilizing ⅛ to ¼ inch trephines and suturing of the superior to inferior edges is often sufficient to correct entropion involving only a portion of the lid (Fig. 43A and B). (2) Excision of an elliptical portion of the lid including a horizontal strip of the underlying orbicularis muscle still remains the most commonly performed and successful procedure. Predetermination of the correct amount of skin to be removed is accomplished by grasping a fold with straight hemostatic forceps, clamping tightly for twenty to thirty seconds, thereby producing a ridge of skin when the forceps is released (Fig. 44A). If the lid margin is

Plate 2.

A. Entropion.
B. Ectropion.
C. Distichiasis with corneal damage.

D. Eversion of the membrane nictitans.
E. Hypertrophy of the membrane nictitans.
F. Blepharitis.

Plate 2

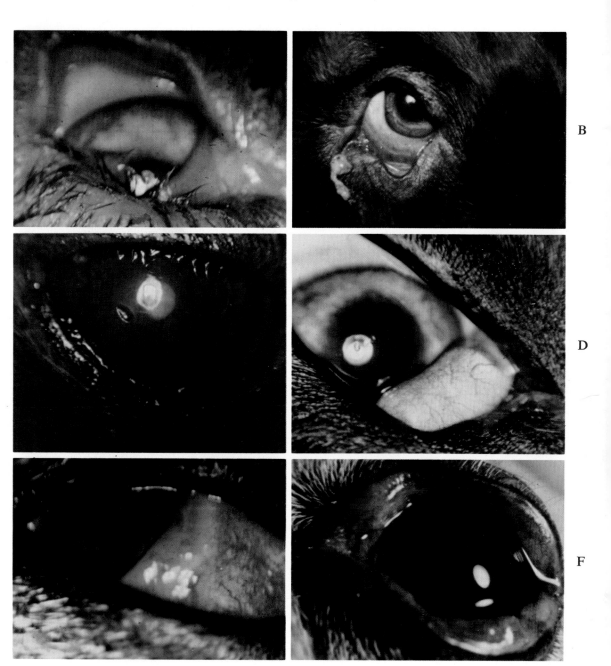

B

D

F

still not in proper proximity to the
globe, the fold can be smoothed out
with the thumb and a bigger or lesser
"bite" taken. When it appears that the
amount of skin is adequate the ridge is
cut at its base with heavy curved scissors (Fig. 44B). This produces a half
moon or elliptical area. Then, commenc-
ing at one end of the wound the orbicularis is elevated with eye tissue forceps
and a strip of muscle removed for the
length of the incision (Fig. 44C). This
step is attended by hemorrhage which
is quickly controlled by the placing of
either interrupted or mattress sutures
through the skin (Fig. 44D). A plastic
collar (Fig. 45A) or plastic pail (Fig.
45B) affords the best protection against
self-injury following any of the lid procedures. Sutures may be removed in
eight to ten days.

4:23　　3. *Canthoplasty* (Par. 4:14)
alone or in combination with skin excision is usually the operation of choice
in those instances where the entropion
results from a narrow palpebral fissure.

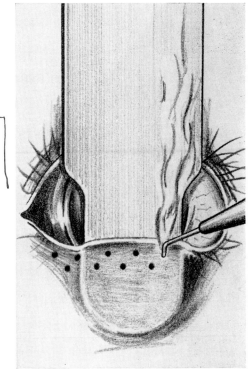

Fig. 42.　Cautery-puncture operation for mild
entropion.

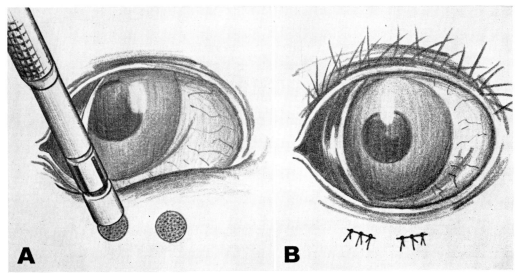

Fig. 43.　Trephine operation for entropion. *A.* Circular areas of skin removed by trephine. *B.* Sutures
placed from superior to inferior edges.

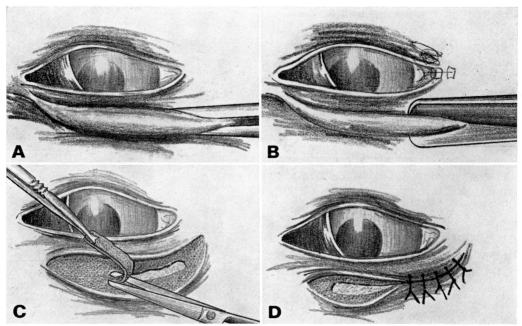

Fig. 44. Surgical correction of entropion. *A*. Ridge of skin is raised by clamping with hemostatic forceps. *B*. The ridge of skin is cut at its base with heavy scissors. *C*. Removing a strip of orbicularis muscle. *D*. Sutures being placed.

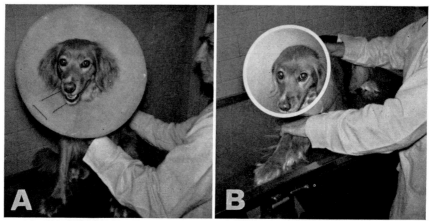

Fig. 45. *A*. Flexible plastic collar in place. *B*. Plastic pail in place.

Ectropion (Plate 2B)

4:24   This is simply an outrolling or eversion of the lid, just the opposite of entropion.

4:25   *Etiology.* The fault is most often congenital and hereditary in the Cocker Spaniel, St. Bernard and Blood Hound breeds. The acquired forms result from cicatricial contraction following accidents or prolonged blepharitis. A senile form results from a relaxing of tissue and lack of tone.

4:26   *Symptoms.* Exposure of conjunctival surface and eversion of the punctum thus causing epiphora (escape of tears) and a reddened, hypertrophied surface. An exposure keratitis may result in the marked cases.

4:27   *Treatment.* 1. Cautery-puncture is effective only in ectropion of limited degree and may need to be repeated. Fixation or lid forceps are clamped on the everted eyelid. The electrocautery or heated muscle hook is thrust through the exposed conjunctiva and muscle in a parallel line about 4 to 5 mm from the lid margin (Fig. 46). About 6 punctures are made and the skin is *not* penetrated. An antibiotic-steroid ointment application several times a day suffices for aftercare.

4:28   2. *Skin excision.* Trephine removal of skin plugs utilizing ⅛ to ¼-inch trephines and suturing the lateral to medial edges is often sufficient to correct the ectropion involving only a portion of the lid (Fig. 47A and B). As an alternative to the trephine method the V-Y technique (Wharton Jones) with or without a canthoplasty (Par. 4:14) is useful, especially in the cicatricial type ectropion. A V-shaped skin incision is made from the lid mar-

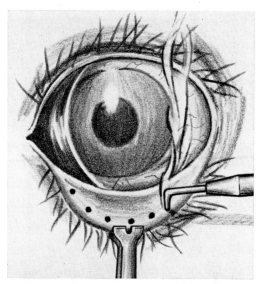

Fig. 46.   Cautery-puncture inside the lid for mild ectropion.

gin, converging at an apex below the involved area (Fig. 48A). The triangle of skin is then undermined with tenotomy scissors in all directions (Fig. 48B). Any subcutaneous scar tissue must be excised. The base of the skin flap remains attached at the lid margin. Beginning at the apex or lowermost part of the V, transverse sutures of 5–0 Dermalon are placed. Additional sutures on

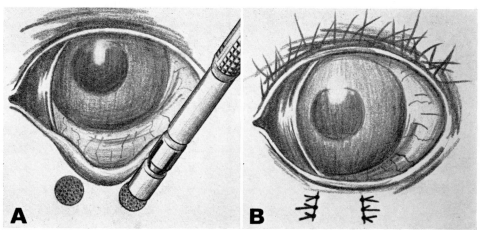

A   **B**

Fig. 47.   Trephine operation for ectropion. A. Circular areas of skin removed by trephine. B. Sutures placed from lateral to medial edges.

either side result in the Y closure, thus raising the lid border to its normal position (Fig. 48C).

4:29   3. *Conjunctival excision.* In those breeds in which an unusual ectropion (Fig. 49A) is responsible for disfigurement or accompanying pathology, the excision of the conjunctiva making up the cul-de-sac (lower transition of bulbar and palpebral conjunc-

tiva) is accomplished in somewhat the reverse fashion as that described for skin excision in the entropion procedure (Par. 4:22). A fold of conjunctival tissue is grasped with straight hemostatic forceps, clamping tightly for twenty to thirty seconds, thereby producing a ridge when the forceps is released (Fig. 49B). The ridge is cut at the base with tenotomy scissors and the opposing wound edges approximated with interrupted

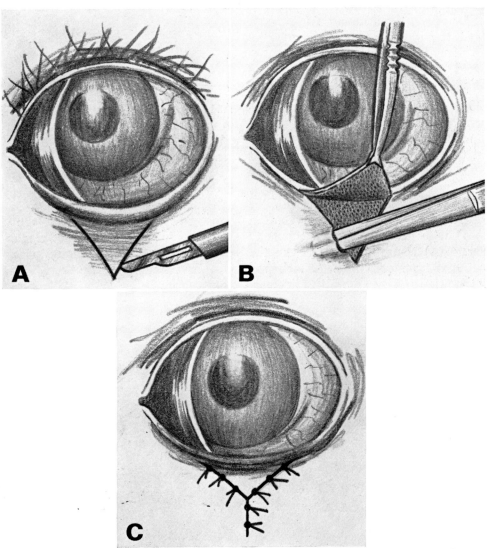

Fig. 48.   Surgical correction of ectropion. *A.* V-shaped skin incision from lid margin. *B.* Undermining of skin. *C.* Resultant Y closure.

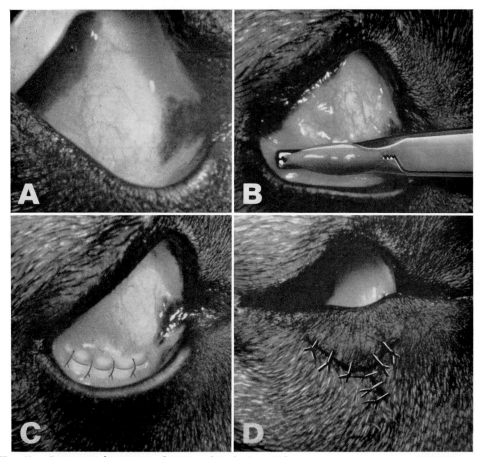

Fig. 49.   Conjunctival excision and V-Y combined. *A.* Initial appearance of ectropion. *B.* Ridge of conjunctiva is raised by clamping with hemostatic forceps.

C. Suture placement following excision of conjunctival ridge. *D.* Final appearance following an additional V-Y operation.

5–0 catgut sutures (Fig. 49C). An additional skin trephine procedure or V-Y operation (Par. 4:28) is often indicated to correct an ectropion of this sort completely (Fig. 49D).

Distichiasis and Trichiasis

4:30   In *distichiasis* a second, abnormal row of eyelashes is present. This row is usually incomplete, with one to a dozen or so lashes arising from the orifices of the meibomian glands. Usually only the upper lid is involved but both may well be (Fig. 50).

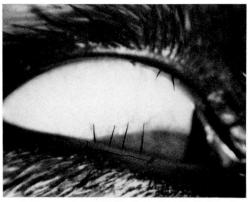

Fig. 50.   Distichiasis involving both upper and lower lids.

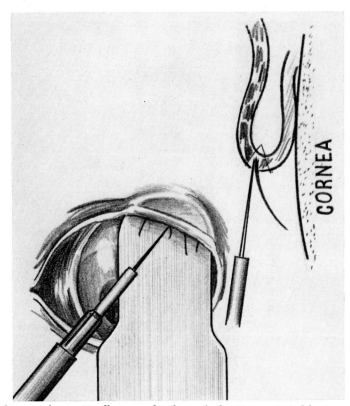

Fig. 51.   Electro-epilation. Needle inserted to base of cilia. Eye protected by tongue depressor.

4:31 *Etiology.* Although considered primarily a congenital condition involving more commonly the Pekingese, Poodle and Bedlington terrier breeds, we have noted that these lashes may occur spontaneously at any age and in any breed.

4:32 *Symptoms.* When the lashes are bristle-like, considerable damage to the conjunctiva and cornea may result (Plate 2C). Epiphora is a most constant accompaniment. Distichiasis is not uncommon to the dog and is often missed because the examiner fails to use magnification in his examination of the orbital structures.

4:33 *Treatment.* Unwanted lashes may be plucked from their orifice or cut flush with the lid margin but this provides only temporary relief. Perma-

nent correction can be achieved by performing electro-epilation (Fig. 51). The Miller-Cameron unit is set on a reading of 1 on the coagulation side. With a special fine epilation needle (Fig. 28B, Chapter 3) the orifice alongside of the lash is entered and the needle inserted to the base of the cilia. The current is turned on as soon as it becomes difficult to insert the needle farther towards the base. Often the cilia will then cling to and be extracted in the withdrawal of the needle. Otherwise, when it is felt that the root has been destroyed, the lash is easily removed with epilation or tissue forceps. The globe is protected by inserting a tape padded tongue depressor between lid and cornea. The owner must be warned that other cilia can appear in new locations at a later date and it is often necessary to perform the procedure a second or third time before all the lashes are destroyed. The procedure is tedious and requires the aid of good magnification.

4:34   A more radical approach (entropion procedure) may be necessary if epilation fails. Removal of a strip of skin and orbicularis muscle suffices to direct the lashes away from the eyeball. However, this naturally results in some disfigurement if no lid anomaly is present and should be reserved as a last resort measure.

4:35   In *trichiasis*, the regular eyelashes assume an abnormal deviation so that they set up a conjunctival or corneal irritation.

4:36   *Etiology.* Sometimes congenital but often the deviation is acquired and is due to a moderate entropion or blepharospasm.

4:37   *Symptoms.* There is epiphora and possible corneal damage (*e.g.* superficial vascularization and scarring) with an accompanying mucoid discharge.

4:38   *Treatment.*   Electro-epilation and/or entropion surgical procedure can be used depending upon the cause.

Diseases and Surgery of the Membrane Nictitans (third eyelid)
(Fig. 52A, B and C)

4:39   At the median aspect of the palpebral aperture is the nictitating membrane, the embedded posterior end of which is surrounded by the *nictitans gland*. Both surfaces of the membrane are covered with epithelium continuous with the bulbar conjunctiva on one side and the palpebral conjunctiva on the other. Within these surfaces lies a plate of hyaline cartilage which is usually "T"

shaped.[2] The plate and surfaces have a concave shape to fit the cornea. The membrane nictitans is well developed in the dog, can be extended over the entire anterior aspect of the globe, and serves the most useful purpose of protecting the eyeball in impending danger. It may also be used advantageously as a conjunctival flap in the surgical correction of several conditions (Par. 5:66).

4:40   *Eversion* of the membrane nictitans occurs as a congenital anomaly in several breeds (*e.g.* Danes, Weimariners). In these instances the cartilage appears to be defective, causing the upper half of the membrane to fold forward on itself (Plate 2D).

4:41   *Symptoms.* These are epiphora or mucoid discharge; disfigurement.

4:42   *Treatment.* The entire membrane may be removed at its base or the folded top portion cut off and the anterior and posterior conjunctival surfaces sutured over the top of the cartilage. However, in order to preserve the integrity of the membrane for cosmetic purposes and retain its protective usefulness, removal of the cartilage and posterior gland structure is easily accomplished and is, by far, the preferable solution.

4:43   The membrane (Fig. 53A) is positioned with forceps at its free borders on the medial and lateral aspects and stretched upwards and out to expose the inner surface (Fig. 53B). With fine tissue forceps and tenotomy scissors the cartilage and gland is undermined from the top to its base and simply cut out (Fig. 53C). This leaves a smooth junctional membrane sans supportive cartilage, which seems unimportant anyway (Fig. 53D).

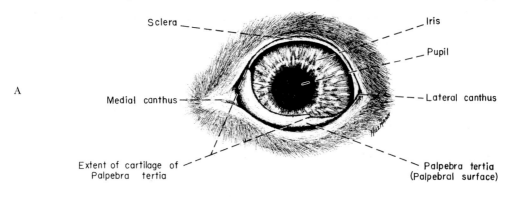

A

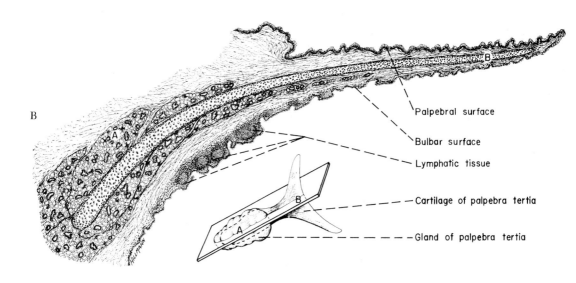

B

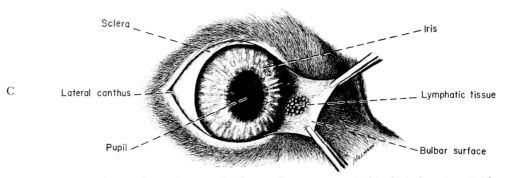

C

Fig. 52.   *A.* The membrane nictitans. *B.* The membrane nictitans in histological section. *C.* The membrane nictitans reflected to reveal lymphatic tissue. (Miller, Christensen and Evans, Anatomy of the Dog, courtesy of W. B. Saunders Company.)

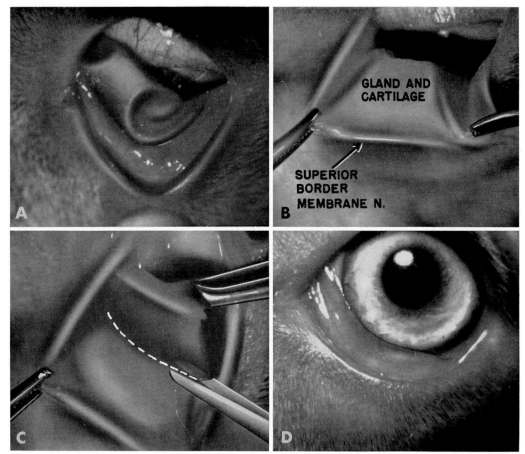

Fig. 53. *A.* Eversion of membrane nictitans. *B.* Membrane positioned and gland and cartilage exposed. *C.* Extirpation of gland and cartilage following undermining. *D.* Immediate postoperative view of corrected eversion.

Hypertrophy of the Membrane Nictitans

4:44 This condition is occasionally encountered in the larger breeds as an inherited anomaly but may be acquired as a chronic inflammatory process. A thickened protruding membrane appears secondary to several diseases of the orbit (Chapter 8) and as an ocular manifestation of malignant lymphoma (Par. 12:35). An embedded foreign body may well be the cause. Thus a careful evaluation of each case is imperative.

4:45 *Symptoms.* The thickened, flushed membrane produces a watery to mucoid discharge. The dog often exhibits discomfort and may rub the eye causing corneal abrasion or infected ulceration. The membrane may remain in a fixed position covering about a third of the eyeball (Plate 2E).

4:46 *Treatment.* The steroid antibiotic combinations are effective when the cause is a specific inflammatory or allergic manifestation. In the event medication fails to alleviate the condition, complete removal of the membrane may be necessary. This is easily accomplished by elevating the superior

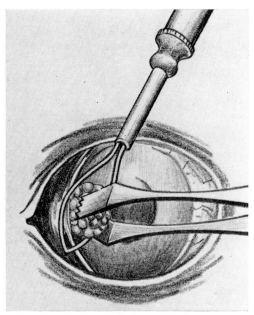

Fig. 54.   Removal of glands of the membrane nictitans with Allis forceps and tonsil snare.

border with fixation forceps and cutting at the base with heavy curved scissors. Since the membrane does serve a useful purpose (Par. 4:39) and its absence can predispose to various keratopathies this procedure should only be performed as a last resort. Neither must congenital eversion of the membrane (Par. 4:40) be confused with hypertrophy since often the structure can be preserved in true eversion.

Hypertrophy of the Nictitans Gland

4:47   This is not considered a congenital anomaly as such but there is a particular breed predisposition to its occurrence in the spaniel and Boston terrier breeds.

4:48   *Symptoms.* The glandular tissue projects beyond the membrane nictitans as a round, red mass often referred to as "cherry" eye. Aside from some excess in tearing and the possible production of a mucoid discharge, it

appears to cause little discomfort to the dog.

4:49   *Treatment.* The use of steroid preparations will often reduce the edematous protrusion but surgical extirpation offers the only permanent means of correction. The glandular tissue may be simply cut out with forceps and scissors (Par. 4:43). A more satisfactory method, offering the advantages of little to no hemorrhage and which can be performed safely under topical anesthesia, is to use Allis forceps and a tonsil snare (Fig. 54).

Atresia

4:50   *Atresia* or congenital absence of the openings to the lacrimal canal is not uncommon, especially to the Bedlington, Sealyham and Poodle breeds. Either or both the upper and lower punctum may be absent or covered by a thin membrane. It is, however, more common to find the inferior opening occluded in this manner.

4:51   *Symptoms.* Epiphora (spillage of tears) producing a rust colored tear streak at the nasal fold is to be expected. Many dogs, however, may go through life with occluded or absent punctae showing little evidence of this "wet eye" anomaly. In these instances a compensatory mechanism apparently results in less actual tear production by the lacrimal gland.

4:52   *Treatment.* It is sometimes possible to re-establish patency of an inferior opening when the punctum is covered by a membrane. By irrigating through the superior opening a ballooning will be noted at the intended origin of the inferior opening (Fig. 55A). This ballooned area is "knicked" or a small piece is cut away, allowing the solution to escape (Fig. 55B). Restoration of the patency of the passage is not always permanent, but daily irrigation (five to seven days) and massage is helpful in discouraging a postoperative closure.

4:53 Complete surgical restoration of the nasolacrimal drainage apparatus by means of a dacryocystorhinostomy and plastic drainage tubes is a most specialized procedure, often important to man's well being, but seldom indicated in the dog.

Epiphora

4:54 Roberts[6] concludes that chronic epiphora in dogs is related not to overproduction of tears, but rather to anatomic defects or functional disturbances that interfere with drainage through the nasal lacrimal canals. This may ordinarily be the case, but irritation of one sort or another will certainly provoke excess tear formation. Once the irritative source is eliminated, the excess tearing stops.

4:55 *Etiology.* Causes include: atresia, plugged ducts, allergens, distichiasis, trichiasis, entropion, ectropion, eversion and/or hypertrophy of the membrane nictitans, and contact with hair from the nasal skin folds and periorbital skin. A peculiar cause of epiphora in poodles (and some Pomeranians) appears to stem from a normal appearing nictitans gland.

4:56 *Treatment.* In the poodle with epiphora and staining of the nasal folds, it has been our practice under general anesthesia to determine the patency of the nasolacrimal drainage apparatus, possible presence of distichiasis, and the lid apposition to the globe. It should be noted that simple instillation of fluorescein dye in the conjunctival sac and awaiting its appearance at the nostril are not always reliable tests as to the

patency of the ducts. Irrigation with saline solution employing a lacrimal canula and syringe will disclose much more information (Fig. 56).

4:57 After "checking out" and discounting these possible causes of epiphora, the nictitans glands are removed

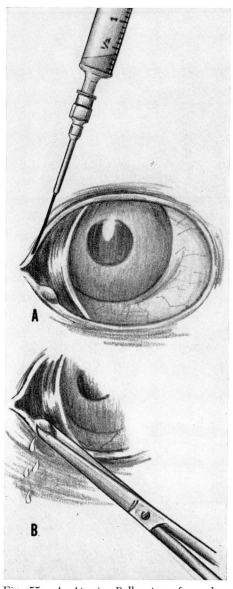

Fig. 55. *A.* Atresia. Ballooning of membrane which covers the opening. *B.* Cutting membrane to correct the atresia.

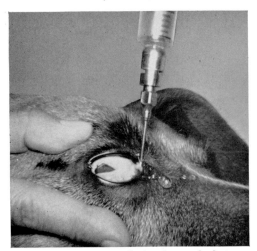

Fig. 56. Irrigation of the lacrimal drainage system.

in one of the manners described (Par. 4:43 and Par. 4:49). In most instances this results in a substantial decrease in tearing and spillage.

Other Lid Diseases

4:58   Other common affections of the eyelids not associated with inheritance or breed predisposition include edema, blepharitis, periorbital dermatitis, chalazion, hordeolum, lid abscess, wounds, foreign bodies, and tumors.

Edema

4:59   *Etiology.* Simple edema of the lids is usually of allergic origin (insect bites, pollen), however, trauma, infection, periorbital dermatitis or demodex mange may be exciting factors.

4:60   *Treatment.* Treatment directed at the cause will usually afford quick relief. Antibiotic-steroid combinations are effective in those cases of allergic or infectious origin. Goodwinol ointment* is a specific for demodex mange of the lids.

* Goodwinol Products Corp., Wappingers Falls, N. Y.

Blepharitis (Plate 2F)

4:61   *Symptoms.* The symptoms are inflammatory edema with reddening and thickening of the palpebral conjunctiva and lid margins, sticky discharge, blepharospasm.

4:62   *Etiology.* Etiology consists of contact with irritating weeds, mange, dermatitis, nutritional deficiencies, association with hordeolum, chalazion, accompanying or following distemper, or in combination with conjunctivitis or keratoconjunctivitis.

4:63   *Sequelae.* Sequelae include hypertrophy of the lid margins, trichiasis, entropion and ectropion.

4:64   *Treatment.* The disease is often obstinate. A determination of the causes and its removal is important. It is well to have the lid hair cut closely. The secretions should be cleansed thoroughly from the conjunctival sac before instillation of an antibiotic-steroid ointment to the outer and inner lid margins. Surgical drainage and curettage (Par. 4:71), or manual expression of the purulent material is often indicated in those instances in which the sebaceous or meibomian glands are involved.

Chalazion

4:65   Chalazion (tarsal cyst) is an inflammatory enlargement of the meibomian glands resulting from stoppage of a duct and accompanied by involvement of the surrounding tissues.

4:66   *Symptoms.* A painless, pea-like swelling in the upper or lower eyelid (Fig. 57). It develops slowly and the contents are usually a cheesy material. When the lid is everted, the conjunctiva over the chalazion is seen to be reddened and elevated. A conjunctival irritation may result or if the chalazion becomes chronic, it may involve the lid margin in the form of a granuloma.

4:67 *Treatment.* Treatment consists of incision and curettage. A chalazion clamp is applied and the eyelid is everted. An incision is made through the conjunctiva over the swelling (Fig. 58A) and the walls of the chalazion thoroughly curetted (Fig. 58B). The clamp is released and an antibiotic ointment applied for several days postoperatively. In the chronic form (granu-

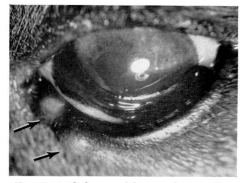

Fig. 57. Chalazion of lower lid. Note the two pea-like swellings.

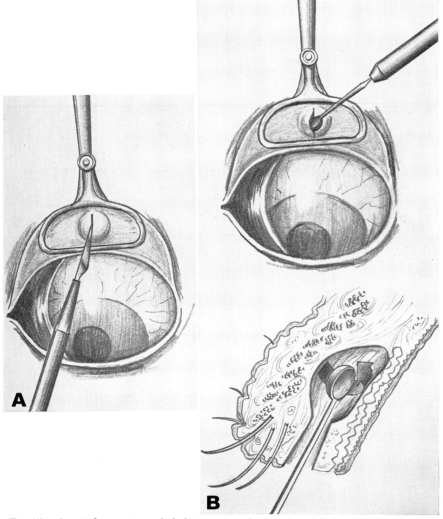

Fig. 58. Surgical correction of chalazion. *A.* Lid everted and incision. *B.* Curettage.

loma), electrocoagulation may be necessary.

Hordeolum

4:68 Hordeolum is a circumscribed, acute inflammation at the edge of the lid resulting from a staphylococcus involvement of the sebaceous glands and cilia.

4:69 *Symptoms.* It is usually painful and apt to provoke a blepharospasm and lacrimation. The condition is frequently associated with a blepharitis and an abscess ordinarily develops.

4:70 *Treatment.* Incision, and application of an antibiotic ointment rubbed thoroughly into the lid margins will usually suffice. If recurrences persist, injections of a staphylococcus toxoid and systemic antibiotics are of value.

Lid Abscess (Fig. 59A)

4:71 Lid abscessation can result from penetrating wounds, embedded foreign bodies, chalazion, hordeolum, or chronic meibomitis. Immediate relief and correction are usually attained by surgical drainage, flushing of the

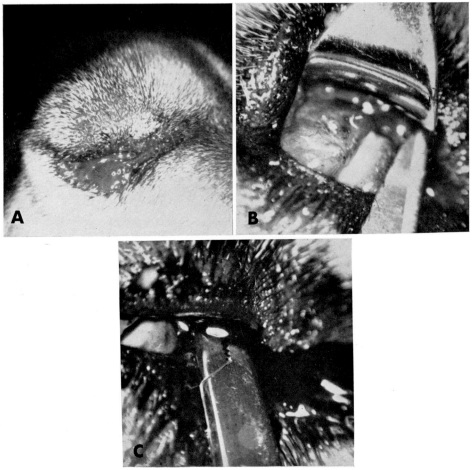

Fig. 59. *A.* Lid abscessation. *B.* Incision into the fornix area with upper lid retracted. *C.* Drainage established by inserting and spreading blades of a mosquito forceps.

abscess sac and the instillation of an antibiotic ointment. Most abscesses involve the upper lid and the fornix offers the best incision site (Fig. 59B). Enlarging of the incision to provide adequate drainage is accomplished by inserting and spreading the blades of the mosquito forceps (Fig. 59C).

Wounds

4:72   Lacerations of the eyelids are not uncommon and result from bites, cat scratches, automobile injuries and entanglement with hooks and wire. These injuries produce a variety of tears, the surgical correction of which often proves a challenge. The possibility of injury to the globe must not be overlooked.

4:73   Wounds should be repaired as soon as possible after injury. The general principles of repair include:
1. Thorough cleansing of the wound and removal of all foreign material.
2. Minimal debridement. Nonviable appearing tissue often may be saved.
3. Eyelid must be sutured in layers. It is important to close the conjunctiva (5–0 chromic catgut) and to repair the orbicularis muscle when needed.
4. The use of fine needles and suture material (5–0 dermalon), immobilization by bandaging, and prevention of self-mutilation by the use of a plastic collar (Fig. 45A) or pail (Fig. 45B) is essential to success.

4:74   In the repair of eyelid wounds with considerable loss of tissue, plastic surgery employing a sliding flap technique is occasionally necessary.

Tumors

4:75   Papillomata (Fig. 60), including verruca (wart), are the most commonly encountered growths. When located on the lid they may be snipped off and a silver nitrate stick applied. If the lid margin is involved and there is danger of notching from excision, electrocautery offers a splendid means of performing safe, bloodless surgery with minimal loss of tissue. More extensive neoplasms (Plate 3F) are always most easily removed by electrocautery. Dermoid cyst (congenital) (Fig. 61) re-

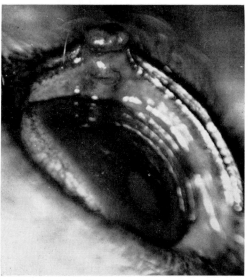

Fig. 60.   Papillomata with deep extension.

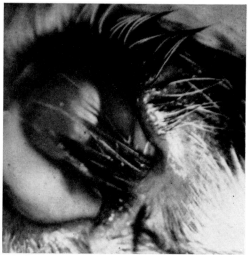

Fig. 61.   Dermoid of the lower lid and lateral canthus.

moval is easily performed by simple excision. The scalpel incisions are made through the skin and down to the underlying bulbar conjunctiva. These upper and lower incisions are made to meet at what should be the lateral canthus (Fig. 62A). The skin and dermoid is then undermined and dissected free of the conjunctiva. The resulting wound is allowed to heal "open" (Fig. 62B).

Infections of the Lacrimal Apparatus

4:76   Occlusion of the lacrimal canal (Par. 4:50) and epiphora (Par. 4:55) has been discussed.

Dacryoadenitis

4:77   Inflammation, abscess formation or new growths in the lacrimal gland (Par. 8:10) is uncommon to the dog. Xerophthalmosis, denoting a condition of the lacrimal gland when it ceases to secrete tears, is frequently encountered on a temporary or permanent basis. Causes include chronic distemper, senility, and injuries to the gland with subsequent degeneration and loss of function (Par. 6:57).

Dacryocystitis

4:78   Inflammation of the lacrimal sac is usually due to an obstruction in the nasolacrimal duct followed by infection of the sac. The condition cannot be considered common in the dog probably because the sac is underdeveloped as compared to man. ***However, it is often the cause of a seemingly obscure unilateral conjunctivitis which fails to respond to any treatment*** (Par. 5:44). The sac serves as a reservoir of infection, continually inoculating the conjunctiva via the inferior lacrimal opening (puncta). Also, because there is no adequate drainage from the sac to the nasolacrimal duct, there remains but this one escape route for the infected discharge.

4:79   *Treatment.* Thorough irrigation (Fig. 56) of the drainage apparatus and establishment of patency, if possible, are important. Instillation of an oily penicillin preparation through the lacrimal needle often suffices to clear up the sac infection.

4:80   In the event medical treatment proves ineffective, surgical extirpation of the sac is indicated. A probe placed in the upper opening and extending to the sac area offers a good landmark for the incision site (Fig. 63). It is difficult

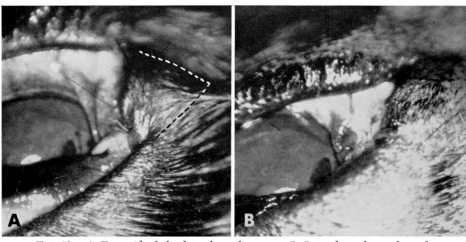

Fig. 62.   A. Dermoid of the lateral canthus area. B. Lateral canthus reformed.

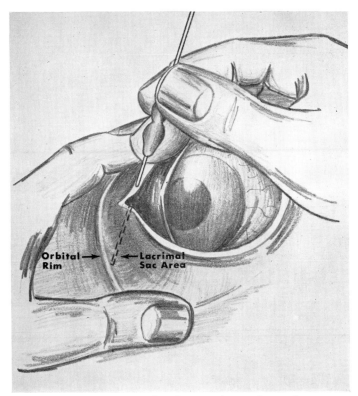

Fig. 63.   Cut away view of probe extending to lacrimal sac area.

to define the actual sac but infected tissue will be found just inside the orbital rim. Its removal by dissection and scraping will ordinarily offer permanent relief.

References

1. Magrane, William G.: Ocular Physiology, No. Am. Vet., *36*, 388, 1955.

2. Prince, Jack H., Diesem, Charles D., Eglitis, Irma and Ruskell, Gordon L.: *Anatomy and Histology of the Eye and Orbit in Domestic Animals,* Springfield, Charles C Thomas, 1960.
3. Berens, Conrad and King, H. J.: *An Atlas of Ophthalmic Surgery,* Philadelphia, J. B. Lippincott Co., p. 42, 1961.
4. Smythe, R. H.: *Veterinary Ophthalmology,* London, Bailliere, Tindall & Cox, p. 194, 1956.
5. Symposium on Granulomatous Diseases—Part I: J.A.V.M.A., *127*, 334, 1955.
6. Roberts, S. R.: Abnormal Tear Secretion in the Dog, Mod. Vet. Practice, *43*, 37, 1962.

Chapter 5

DISEASES AND SURGERY OF THE CONJUNCTIVA

Anatomy and Physiology

5:1   The conjunctiva is a thin, transparent mucous membrane lining the inner surface of the lids (*palpebral conjunctiva*) and the anterior surface of the eyeball to the cornea (*bulbar conjunctiva*).

5:2   The palpebral conjunctiva consists of a collagenous lamina propria and a stratified epithelium.[1] It is closely adherent to the underlying tarsus. The area of reflection and transition of palpebral conjunctiva to bulbar conjunctiva is referred to as the *fornix.* The fornix area is loosely folded permitting free rotations of the globe. It is within this area that the ducts from the lacrimal and auxiliary glands discharge their secretions (Par. 4:3).

5:3   The bulbar conjunctiva is loosely attached to the sclera by connective tissue (*episcleral tissue*) except at the corneal-scleral junction (*limbus*) where it is firmly adherent. It continues uninterruptedly over the cornea, becoming the corneal epithelium. Near the inner canthus the conjunctiva extends over a plate of hyaline cartilage (*membrane nictitans* Par. 4:39). *Tenon's capsule* (Par. 1:16) is attached to the globe behind the limbal attachment of the conjunctiva.[2] It surrounds most of the eye and its muscles as a dense connective tissue and lies between the bulbar conjunctiva and episcleral tissue. Because of the close apposition of the bulbar conjunctiva, Tenon's capsule, and the episclera in the perilimbal region, it becomes difficult to dissect down to the sclera in this area (Par. 6:156).

5:4   The bulbar conjunctiva often contains considerable pigment, varying in amount in breeds and individuals. The pigmentation is heaviest at the limbus and proliferation of the limbal

72

melanoblasts into the cornea under certain circumstances causes pigmentary keratitis in the dog (Par. 6:61).

5:5   The substantia propria of the conjunctiva is composed of two layers, a superficial adenoid layer, which in the dog contains lymphatic follicles and glands, and a deep fibrous layer. The nerves and vessels of the conjunctiva are in the fibrous layer.[3]

5:6   The arteries of the conjunctiva come from: 1, the peripheral arterial arcades; 2, the marginal arterial arcades, and 3, the anterior ciliary arteries. The peripheral arcade lies at the upper border of the lid and supplies most of the conjunctiva. These arterial systems all anastomose with each other, forming a large vascular network. The conjunctival veins accompany the arteries but are more numerous. There is a venous plexus similar to the arterial system.

5:7   The lymphatics of the conjunctiva are arranged in a superficial and deep plexus. The lymphatic drainage is towards the commissures, where they join the lymphatics of the lids. The drainage towards the external commissure goes to the parotid nodes, while to the inner side it goes to the submaxillary lymph glands.

5:8   The nerve supply of the conjunctiva is derived from the same source as that of the lids. The anterior ciliaries (branches of the long and short ciliary nerves) that form a plexus in the ciliary body supply the cornea and circumcorneal zone of the conjunctiva, and the lacrimal and infratrochlear supply a much larger area of the conjunctiva than of skin.

Physical States or Changes in the Conjunctiva

5:9   The   conjunctiva   undergoes changes which can be associated with local or systemic pathology.

5:10   1. *Active hyperemia.* The eye appears red and the patient exhibits discomfort (irritative, itchy condition). The causes may include a mechanical or chemical irritation, allergens, or result from, for example, a respiratory infection.

5:11   2. *Passive hyperemia.* The conjunctival vessels appear darker. This usually is an indication of more deep-seated trouble, *i.e.*, an intraocular inflammation.

5:12   3. *Anemia* gives rise to a pale pink conjunctiva and pearly white sclera. This is a good indicator of the systemic state of the patient and calls for further investigation.

5:13   4. *Chemosis* is an edematous swelling of the bulbar conjunctiva (Plate 3A). It results from allergens, local irritants, drug sensitivity (Par. 3:36), conjunctival inflammations and exophthalmos (Par. 8:17).

5:14   5. *Ecchymosis* is characterized by intraconjunctival and subconjunctival hemorrhages and is often seen after injuries, operations and inflammations of the eyeball. The hemorrhage is of no importance and the blood becomes absorbed within a week or two. The disappearance of the discoloration can, however, be materially hastened by using steroids in subconjunctival injection form.[4]

5:15   6. *Follicles* are often present as primarily a lymphoid reaction and usually are part of a chronic inflammatory picture. They may occur simply as the result of allergens and in these instances epiphora can be expected (Par. 4:55).

Conjunctival and Ciliary Injection

5:16   Differential diagnosis between:

Conjunctival Injection	*Ciliary Injection*
1. Conjunctiva involved	1. Cornea, iris, ciliary body and sclera involved
2. Blood vessels injected toward cul-de-sac and fornix	2. Injected at and near limbus
3. Vessels appear bright red	3. Darker
4. Vessels dilated and tortuous	4. Small and straight
5. Vessels can be moved by pressure	5. Vessels not movable
6. $\frac{1}{1000}$ epinephrine will clear	6. Epinephrine without effect
7. Mucoid, mucopurulent or purulent discharge	7. Increased tearing (epiphora)
8. Itching sensation	8. True pain
9. Lids glued in morning	9. Not usually
10. Cornea clear after irrigation	10. Corneal deposits or edema make cornea dull
11. Pupil normal	11. Pupil dilated or constricted
12. Lens and vitreous clear	12. Often not clear
13. Intraocular tension normal	13. Often abnormal—increased or decreased

Congenital Anomalies

5:17   *Dermoid* cyst, a congenital tumor, may involve conjunctiva alone as a mass beneath the skin of the lateral canthus (Fig. 62A). Excision of the mass is easily performed, thus reforming the canthus (Fig. 62B). Or, the dermoid may be situated partially in the conjunctiva and extend over the superficial corneal structures (Plate 4A). In these instances an incision is made down to the sclera opposite the border of the dermoid. Then, by undermining, the dermoid can be easily "peeled off" in the manner of performing a superficial keratectomy (Par. 6:153). Aftercare consists of the instillation of an antibiotic preparation for several days. Re-epithelialization is usually complete within ten to fourteen days.

Conjunctivitis—General Considerations

5:18   Because of its exposed position the conjunctiva comes in contact with more microorganisms than any other mucous membrane.[5] Thus, conjunctivitis is the commonest of all eye diseases encountered. It is well, however, to rule out an accompanying keratitis, glaucoma and iritis as the conjunctival changes are marked and may be misleading in these diseases.

5:19   In general most of the cases of conjunctivitis are caused by bacterial or virus infection, contact allergens, irritation from foreign bodies or chemical substances and trauma. An etiologic diagnosis is not always easy to come by. Often distinctive clinical signs which are diagnostic in the early stages of a disease have disappeared by the time the dog is presented for treatment. In these instances the clinical examination must be supplemented with laboratory studies if the etiology of the condition is to be determined.

5:20   The use of conjunctival scrapings and smears as an aid in diagnosis and treatment has been well documented by Cello.[6] Smears are samples of the exudate found in the conjunctival sac, while scrapings are really limited biopsies in which cells of the living conjunctiva are removed and examined. In preparing a scraping, a small platinum spatula is held at right angles to the conjunctiva and drawn over the surface lightly enough to avoid bleeding, but firmly enough to contact the epithelium. It is convenient to combine smears and scrapings on different sections of the same slide.

5:21 Two slides are prepared so that both a Gram stain and a Giemsa stain can be made. Cello[6] emphasizes the importance of having a standardized method of making the Giemsa preparation since the stain is very sensitive and it is possible to get wide color variations on scrapings from the same eye if the time, concentration, or pH of the stain is changed. Since color differences are used as criteria for degenerative changes, technical errors can lead to false interpretations. A method which has proved satisfactory is as follows:
1. Fix the smear in acetone-free methyl alcohol for fifteen minutes.
2. Flood the smear with stain which has been prepared by adding 1 drop of the Giemsa stock solution to each cc. of glass distilled water (pH 7.0–7.1). Stain for one hour.
3. Decolorize in 95 per cent alcohol for five seconds.
4. Air dry and examine.

5:22 The slides are examined for the presence, number and type of bacteria, changes in the epithelial cells, and number and type of leukocytes. Bacteria are rarely seen in scrapings taken from normal conjunctiva and infrequently in smears made from secretions found in the sac. This is in contrast to surveys where cultural studies revealed a very small percentage of sterile eyes.[6-8] Cello[6] believes that these apparent discrepancies might be explained on the basis of very small numbers of bacteria existing in the healthy conjunctival sac.

5:23 In conjunctivitis, smears and scrapings show an increased number of bacteria, epithelial changes, and an infiltration of leukocytes with or without tissue cells. Scrapings most frequently show only one type of organism and are more accurate than are cultures and smears as a means of determining the bacterium most likely to be primarily involved in the infection.

5:24 Conjunctival scrapings also enable the clinician to evaluate results of treatment. The presence of keratinized cells, goblet cells, bacteria, and leukocytes in an eye which has been under treatment indicates a need for a change in therapy. This is particularly true in infections which show frequent remissions and exacerbations.

5:25 Smear and scraping studies may be supplemented with antibiotic sensitivity tests. Or, the antibiotic sensitivity test alone is often of real value to the busy clinician who has only to:
1. Secure secretions from the conjunctival sac with a sterile cotton applicator.
2. Inoculate brain-heart infusion and incubate for twenty-four to forty-eight hours.
3. Plate out on sensitivity agar with prepared sensitivity discs and read twenty-four hours later.

5:26 A minimum of equipment is needed for this determination and it becomes a practical test from the standpoint of time consumption and economics. Early knowledge of which antibiotic is best suited for alleviation of the condition eliminates the oft expensive trial and error method so distasteful to client, patient, and clinician alike.

5:27 In recent years long continued use of steroid-antibiotic combinations has led to the growth of various fungi in the conjunctival sac. Thus, the use of mycological culture media is sometimes indicated. At the same time these media are inoculated, a check for *Candida albicans* can be made (Pagano-Levin medium*).

* E. R. Squibb, New York, N. Y.

Clinical Types of Conjunctivitis

5:28   Many involved classification systems for diseases of the conjunctiva have been suggested but for the sake of practical simplicity, I offer the following:

1. Acute catarrhal
2. Chronic catarrhal
3. Acute purulent
4. Chronic purulent
5. Special types (secondary)
   A. Lacrimal
   B. Meibomian glands
   C. Keratoconjunctivitis sicca
   D. Endogenous
   E. Allergic
   F. Parasitic
6. Follicular
7. Ophthalmia neonatorum.

Acute Catarrhal Conjunctivitis

5:29   Under this heading belongs inflammations which have a comparatively mild and rapid course and are characterized by the exudation of fluid rather than cellular elements into the conjunctiva, and only rarely do they lead to complications. There is vascular injection and congestion with pinkish to red coloration and a grayish white mucoid to mucopurulent discharge in clots, strings or liquid form. The lids may be swollen and raw. In severe cases there may be added edema of the conjunctiva (chemosis, Par. 5:13). Other symptoms include increased lacrimation and, occasionally, some photophobia. The affection may be limited to one eye, but usually both eyes are implicated, either from the start or after two or three days.

5:30   *Etiology.* The causes are extremely varied. The catarrhal symptoms may be associated with:

    a. Respiratory infection, *e.g.* distemper
    b. Mechanical (entropion, ectro-pion, distichiasis, skin disease of the lids, dogs that ride with their head out the window, and those confined to dusty wind swept runs or are housed on dirty, dusty straw).
    c. Allergy (allergens from grasses and weeds, reaction to long continued use of certain drugs (*e.g.* atropine, dionine), exposure to ultraviolet lights, snowblindness).
    d. Special types of conjunctivitis (Par. 5:44–5:50).
    e. Infections. Bacteria may be the cause, or may play a secondary role in the inflammatory process.

5:31   *Treatment.* Although in many instances the symptoms will abate without interference, treatment reduces the duration, adds to the patient's comfort, and prevents the change into subacute or chronic conjunctivitis. Elimination of the cause is the first consideration, but to determine and eliminate the cause often requires careful questioning of the owner as regards the dog's possible recent exposure.

5:32   The conjunctival sac should be irrigated several times daily with a soothing, antiseptic wash (Par. 3:11) and a bland ointment or castor oil or cod liver oil drops used as a follow-up. In those cases associated with allergens, steroid or steroid-antihistamine preparations are in order (Par. 3:85). When the catarrhal symptoms result from infection, antibiotics with or without steroids or sulfa compounds must be utilized.

Chronic Catarrhal Conjunctivitis

5:33   The chronic catarrhal inflammation presents somewhat similar symptoms to those found in the acute form but is milder in degree. The conjunctiva, especially the palpebral, may be hypertrophied and velvety.

5:34 *Etiology.* The possible causes do not differ from the acute form but in general there is always a bacterial component. The bacterial involvement may be secondary to the primary cause, but nevertheless is present and must be taken into consideration. When the catarrhal form of conjunctivitis becomes chronic, one must investigate the possible causes further, keeping in mind those listed for the acute type, and, in addition, the Special Types (secondary) (Par. 5:44–5:50).

5:35 *Treatment* is essentially that recommended for the acute form except, to achieve the best result, copper sulfate crystal cautery of both the palpebral and bulbar conjunctival surfaces (including the membrane nictitans) with immediate irrigation should precede the use of ophthalmic drops or ointment.

5:36 Copper sulfate cautery (Fig. 64) is easily and safely performed under either topical or short acting general anesthesia.
1. Irrigate all secretions from the sac and dry the surfaces with a cotton applicator.

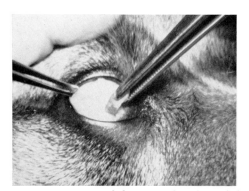

Fig. 64.   Cautery of the external surface of the membrane nictitans with a copper sulfate crystal.

2. Grasp the superior border of the membrane nictitans with fixation forceps and extend it perpendicularly.
3. A smoothed copper sulfate crystal is held with thumb forceps in the opposite hand and is rubbed lightly; first in the lower conjunctival cul-de-sac and on the anterior surface of the membrane nictitans, thence around the undersurface of the lids (palpebral conjunctiva), the superior bulbar conjunctiva and, finally, the inner, glandular surface of the membrane nictitans (membrane now held towards the operator).
4. An assistant irrigates immediately and before the membrane nictitans is released to assume its normal position on the lower globe. This procedure neutralizes the cauterant and prevents any from coming in contact with the cornea.

Acute Purulent Conjunctivitis

5:37 In this type all symptoms of catarrhal conjunctivitis are exaggerated. There is a heavier, thicker discharge, and, in most instances, there is a corneal involvement. Cultures and antibiotic sensitivity tests are of value because this type of conjunctivitis always has its bacterial component. Hemolytic and non-hemolytic *Staphylococcus albus*, *Staphylococcus aureus*, and hemolytic and non-hemolytic streptococci have been found to be the principal organisms involved.[9, 10]

5:38 *Treatment* again consists of repeated irrigations (Par. 3:4) and the use of the antibiotic agent specific for the organisms involved. The clinician should watch for extensive corneal or intraocular complications. In the event this condition is unilateral, attention must be given to the possibility that an embedded foreign body behind the membrane nictitans or a dacryocystitis (Par. 4:78) is responsible.

Chronic Purulent Conjunctivitis

5:39   Chronic purulent conjunctivitis is one of the most refractory conditions we have to cope with in a consideration of diseases of the eye.[11] Pathologically it is characterized by conjunctival hyperemia and a subepithelial reaction consisting of fibrin and edema plus polymorphonuclear leukocytes, lymphocytes, and plasma cells. Certain organisms tend to provoke specific tissue responses, such as follicles, membranes, and ulcers.

5:40   The nature of the discharge causes excoriation, the lids tend to stick together, and the hair surrounding the lids mats up. Corneal involvement ranging from a simple superficial vascularization to deep ulceration is a distinct possibility. Pigmentary keratitis (Par. 6:63) will be a sequela to the stress created by the chronic discharge.

5:41   *Etiology.* Any cause of catarrhal conjunctivitis must be considered. It is essential that every effort be expended to find possible foci of infection. Infections of the ear, skin, and anal sacs occasionally go hand in hand with this chronic type of conjunctivitis. If but one eye is involved a secondary source must be considered (Par. 5:44).

5:42   *Treatment.* Even when culture and antibiotic sensitivity tests suggest the use of specific antibiotics, the attempts to clear the infection are often frustrating. Chronic tissue changes may be so extensive as to interfere with absorption of the antibiotic. It is definitely known that many of the infecting organisms flourish in the subepithelial tissues—beyond reach, so to speak.[11] It is therefore most important that copper sulfate cautery (Par. 5:36) should precede the application of an ophthalmic antibiotic agent. This sloughing of the epithelial layer thus allows a better penetration of the drug.

5:43   A favorable response to this combined chemical cautery and the use of a specific antibiotic or antibiotic-sulfa combination is often followed by a relapse and return of the discharge a week or so later.

Secondary Types of Conjunctivitis

A. Lacrimal

5:44   In this condition the conjunctiva is infected secondarily to infection or blockage of the nasolacrimal tract (dacryocystitis) (Par. 4:78). It is often *unilateral* and the cause is easily overlooked unless an exploration of the lacrimal sac area is made (Par. 4:2). The conjunctivitis responds well to treatment once the reservoir of infection is eliminated (Par. 4:79).

B. Meibomian Glands

5:45   Infection of the Meibomian glands (meibomitis) can lead to a chronic low grade conjunctivitis. In these instances infected material can be expressed from the glands by placing a tongue depressor under the lid and applying downward pressure with the thumb. If the glands become severely involved, *i.e.*, multiple chalazia (Par. 4:65) or lid abscess (Par. 4:71), more extensive treatment is needed.

Plate 3.
A. Chemosis.
B. Chronic purulent conjunctivitis.
C. Follicles on the external surface of the membrane nictitans.
D. Conjunctival hyperplasia encroaching onto the cornea.
E. Verruca of the bulbar conjunctiva.
F. Neoplasm involving the lid and conjunctiva.

Plate 3

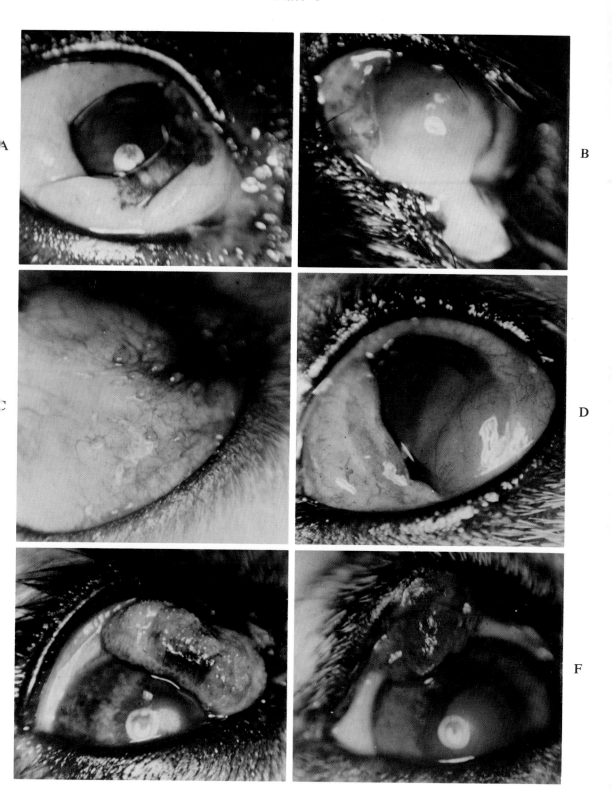

C. *Keratoconjunctivitis Sicca*

5:46   A deficiency of tears and pre-corneal film production leads to a chronic, catarrhal conjunctivitis with a sticky, stringy discharge clinging to a hypertrophied and velvety conjunctiva. This condition, too, is more often *unilateral* and the conjunctivitis will not respond to treatment unless artificial tear therapy is instituted. Since the cornea is always affected, a more thorough discussion of this disease is found in Chapter 6 (Par. 6:55–6:58).

D. *Endogenous*

5:47   A conjunctival discharge may result from a toxic effect from organisms or a true metastasis of the organism from the body to the eye in a systemic infection.

E. *Allergic*

5:48   A mild, non-specific conjunctival inflammation is commonly associated with hay fever. In addition, a larger group of cases of conjunctivitis is due to an allergic reaction to other pollens, dust, bacteria, fungi, ultraviolet light, and topical eye medicaments. Clinical findings include itching, mild photophobia and epiphora. Follicle formation on the bulbar conjunctiva (especially the membrane nictitans) can be expected.

5:49   Elimination of the offending allergens is the most effective treatment. Aside from this, symptomatic treatment with topical steroids or steroid-antihistamine preparations will give relief.

F. *Parasitic*

5:50   A parasite peculiar to the West Coast states, *Thelazia californiensis*, is occasionally observed in the conjunctival cul-de-sac[12, 13] (Fig. 65). Lacrimation and exudation with possible corneal involvement can be expected. No information regarding the intermediate host or vector of this parasite is available, although it has been reported to be transmitted by flies in other parts of the world. Treatment consists of manual removal of the parasites.

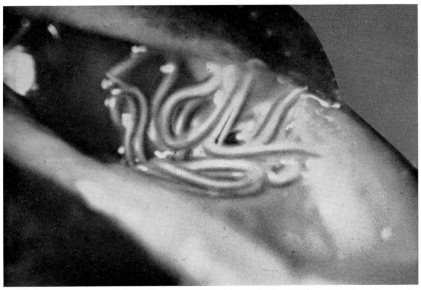

Fig. 65.   Thelazia in the medial canthus area. (Courtesy of Dr. William Zontine, Lancaster, Cal.)

Follicular

5:51   This condition is characterized by the formation of "follicles," with or without the symptoms of catarrhal conjunctivitis.

5:52   A. *Mild.* Small follicles can be seen (with magnification) on the bulbar conjunctiva including the anterior and posterior surfaces of the membrane nictitans. Allergens and mechanical irritation (wind, dust) are the usual causes. Epiphora is to be expected. Elimination of the cause and instillation of any soothing ophthalmic preparation is sufficient.

5:53   B. *Chronic.* This form is accompanied by the chronic catarrhal or purulent forms of conjunctivitis with proliferation of conjunctival tissue. Copper sulfate cautery (Par. 5:36) is essential to the treatment. The follicles are thus sloughed off and the conjunctiva prepared for the subsequent instillation of the ophthalmic preparation indicated.

Ophthalmia Neonatorum

5:54   An acute purulent conjunctivitis occurs in the newborn puppy before lid separation takes place. The lid area appears swollen and an exudate is soon noted extruding from a small lid opening (Fig. 66A). Both eyes are usually involved. If the condition is not recognized early or left untreated, severe corneal involvement may result with a subsequent iris prolapse and loss of an eye.

5:55   *Treatment.* It is imperative that, on noting the first symptoms, a lid separation is performed. This is easily accomplished with the blunt tenotomy scissors (Fig. 66B). By thus exposing the conjunctival surfaces and globe, topical antibiotic therapy can be insti-

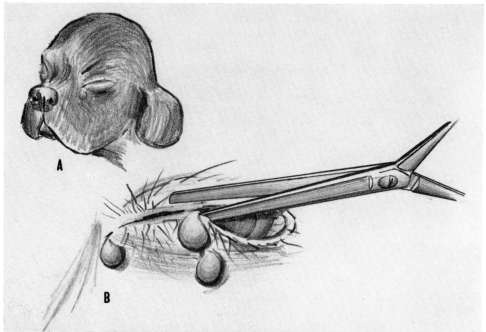

Fig. 66.   *A.* Ophthalmia neonatorum. Discharge seeping from behind closed lids. *B.* Separation of the lids with blunt tenotomy scissors.

tuted. The prognosis then is generally favorable.

Surgical Diseases of the Conjunctiva
Inflammatory Hyperplasia

5:56 An apparent allergen-producing inflammatory process resembling pterygium of man results in a conjunctival encroachment and overgrowth onto the cornea.

5:57 *Treatment.* In the early stages use of the steroids by subconjunctival injection (Par. 3:56) and topical instillation will cause regression and clearing. If there is considerable corneal involvement (Fig. 67 and Plate 3D), a superficial keratectomy is indicated (Par. 6:152). It may be necessary to continue steroids indefinitely to prevent recurrence.

Tumors (Plate 3E, F)

5:58 Tumors of the conjunctiva include dermoids (Par. 5:17) and papilloma (Fig. 68) as more common growths. Malignant tumors are rare but an extension of an intraocular melanoma is possible and would require

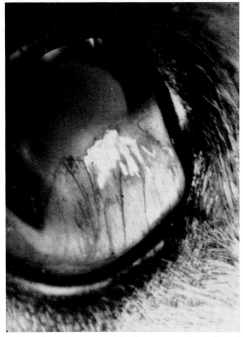

Fig. 67. Pterygium-like lesion invading the superficial cornea.

enucleation or exenteration of the orbit.

Injuries

These are fairly common and include:

5:59 1. *Foreign bodies* are found in

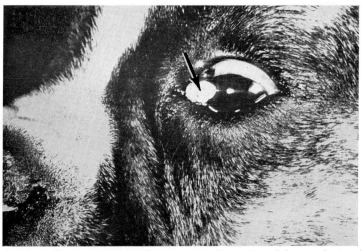

Fig. 68. Viral oral papilloma growing on the conjunctival covering of the membrane nictitans. (Courtesy of Dr. Wayne H. Riser, Philadelphia, Pa.)

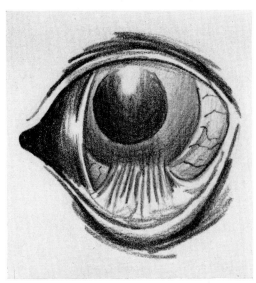

Fig. 69.   Symblepharon (adhesion of bulbar to palpebral conjunctiva).

the conjunctival cul-de-sac or behind the membrane nictitans. These usually consist of weed seeds and awns which, in turn, can cause a corneal involvement. A unilateral conjunctival discharge with accompanying irritative symptoms is suggestive of an embedded foreign body. The majority of these are easily removed following instillation of a topical anesthetic and exposure of the area by elevating the superior border of the membrane nictitans (Par. 2:17).

5:60   2. *Wounds.* Simple tears in the conjunctiva need not be sutured but the clinician is cautioned to examine the area and globe carefully to be certain the laceration is not the site of entry for an embedded foreign body. Extensive conjunctival lacerations should be closed with 5–0 chromic catgut after carefully examining the underlying structures.

5:61   3. *Burns* due to hot liquids, lime, chemicals, soap and detergents

may leave a granulating surface which heals by cicatrization. A *symblepharon* (adhesion of bulbar to palpebral conjunctiva) can result (Fig. 69). A symblepharon may limit the size of the cul-de-sac or interfere with rotation of the eye. If the adhesion area is not too large, it can be severed. Then, by using massage and several daily instillations of an ophthalmic ointment to prevent re-adhesion, it is allowed to fill in gradually.

5:62   But if the symblepharon is extensive and the resulting contraction of the conjunctiva is pronounced, a graft may be necessary. The graft material best suited for conjunctival replacement is the buccal mucosa.

5:63   The first step in the repair of an eye in this condition (symblepharon) is to loosen and dissect away the scarred and vascularized tissue from the underlying sclera until the globe rotates freely. The defect is then lined with a thin graft of buccal mucous membrane. The graft is sutured to the adjacent

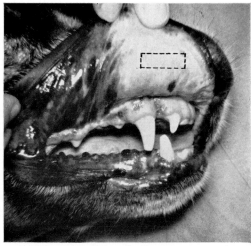

Fig. 70.   Area from which a mucous membrane graft may be obtained.

conjunctiva with interrupted 5–0 catgut, all stitches being *anchored* to the sclera to prevent contraction of the graft.

5:64 The graft is easily obtained from inside the lip or from the gum (Fig. 70). The graft should be scraped and thinned down enough so that it consists only of epithelium and a minimum of supporting tissue.[14] Preparation and use of a graft in this manner may also be indicated in instances in which there is extensive loss of conjunctiva, *e.g.,* wounds or following new growth removal.

Conjunctival Flap Surgery

5:65 The preparation of and uses for the conjunctival flap will be discussed in this chapter since the procedure does constitute conjunctival surgery. The conjunctiva as such, or in the form of conjunctival flaps of various forms, is an invaluable means for the correction of various pathological conditions of the globe which undoubtedly would result in the loss of the globe were not this means available.[15]

5:66 There are many conventional methods of separating the conjunctiva from the sclera and stretching it over a part or all of the cornea to cover a lesion. It becomes necessary in man to utilize the bulbar conjunctiva as such, but the veterinary surgeon has a real advantage in this respect in that the well-developed membrane nictitans of the dog can be used. The advantages over the conventional methods are:
a. The procedure is more easily performed than the regular conjunctival flap operation.
b. The globe itself can be immobilized.
c. The procedure can be used for the same purposes:

1. In an impending iris prolapse (deep ulceration) (Par. 6:107).
2. Following an iris prolapse (after the iris has been snipped off flush with the cornea) (Par. 6:116).
3. To bring a blood supply to a non-healing ulcerous area. The inner surface of the membrane is first scarified.
4. In bullous keratitis (Par. 6:54).
5. In corneal wounds that cannot be opposed perfectly by sutures (Par. 6:125).

5:67 This is an especially useful operation in short-nosed breeds where snug bandaging (which might serve the same purpose) is difficult to achieve. Mechanical support for the eye is obtained through the pressure immobilization provided by this technique.

Technique

5:68 Instrument requirements: two double armed sutures (*e.g.,* Vetafil), needle forceps, eye fixation forceps (Graefe), knife blade (if scarifing indicated).

5:69 Two mattress sutures are placed through the superior edge of the nictitans at its medial and lateral aspects (Fig. 71A). The needle must penetrate both surfaces of the membrane to incorporate the cartilage. The needles are then brought through the upper conjunctival fornix area to the outside skin (Fig. 71B). The membrane is then pulled up snug over the eyeball and the sutures tied down over buttons for better retention and to prevent pressure necrosis (Fig. 71C and D). The globe is now fully enveloped and immobilized by the membrane nictitans and the sutures are not in contact with the corneal surface.

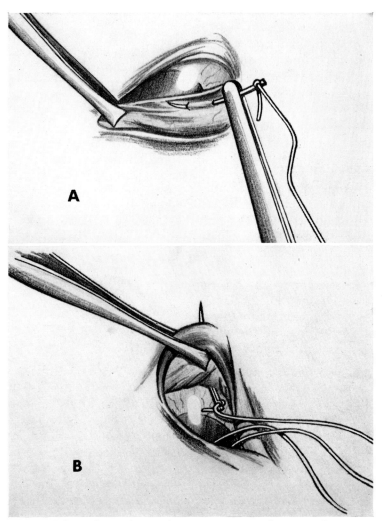

Fig. 71.   Conjunctival flap utilizing the membrane nictitans. *A.* Placement of sutures in the nictitans.
B. Needle through the fornix to the outside skin.

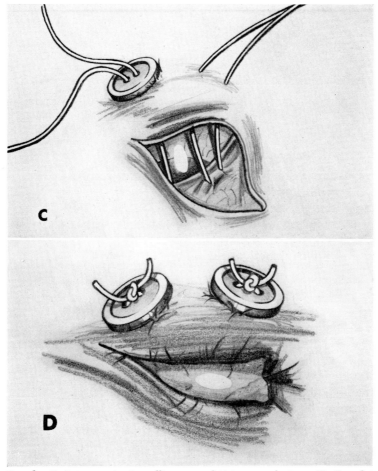

Fig. 71 *continued.* C. Sutures prior to pulling up and tieing over buttons. D. Completed operation.

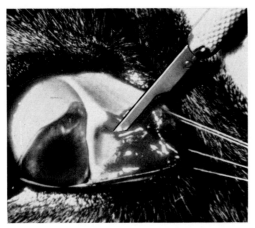

Fig. 72.   Scarifying inner glandular surface of the membrane nictitans. Note pre-placed sutures.

5:70   If scarifying is indicated (Fig. 72), this is done just prior to the pulling up of the membrane. Depending upon the nature of the case, it may be advantageous to remove completely the glands of the nictitans (Par. 4:49) before utilizing it as a conjunctival flap.

5:71   The sutures are left in place for one week. During this time, the eye can be cleansed and medication used through the partial lid opening (Fig. 71D). If the membrane has been scarified, it may remain adhered to the ulcerous cornea following suture removal. This will usually pull loose of its own within a few hours to a day, but can be separated with a smooth spatula if necessary.

References

1. Trautman, Alfred and Fiebiger, Josef: *Fundamentals of the Histology of Domestic Animals*, 8th and 9th ed., Ithaca, Comstock Publishing Associates, p. 405, 1952.
2. Prince, Jack H., Diesem, Charles D., Eglitis, Irma and Ruskell, Gordon L.: *Anatomy and Histology of the Eye and Orbit in Domestic Animals*, Springfield, Charles C Thomas, p. 45, 1960.
3. Cello, Robert M., Krawitz, Leonard and Magrane, William G.: Anatomy Notes, Home Study Course, Am. Soc. of Vet. Ophthal.
4. Magrane, William G.: Cortisone in Ophthalmology, No. Am. Vet., *32*, 763, 1951.
5. Vaughan, D., Cook, R. and Asbury, T.: *General Ophthalmology*, 3rd ed., Los Altos, Lange Medical Publications, 1962.
6. Cello, Robert M.: The Use of Conjunctival Scrapings in the Diagnosis and Treatment of External Diseases of the Eye, Gaines Vet. Symp., Oct. 24, 1956.
7. Jones, G. W.: A Preliminary Report of the Flora in Health and Disease of the External Ear and Conjunctival Sac of the Dog, J.A.V.M.A., *127*, 443, 1955.
8. Correa, W. M. *et al.*: Canine Conjunctivitis, J.A.V.M.A., *138*, 503, 1961.
9. Magrane, William G.: An Evaluation of the Use of Antibiotics in Canine Ophthalmology, No. Am. Vet., *32*, 169, 1951.
10. Magrane, William G.: The Clinical Use of Chloromycetin in Canine Ocular Infections, No. Am. Vet., *34*, 39, 1953.
11. *Canine Medicine*, 2nd ed., Santa Barbara, American Veterinary Publications, Inc., p. 519, 1959.
12. Allerton, F. R.: Worm Parasites on Conjunctivae in Dogs, No. Am. Vet., *10*, 56, 1929.
13. Knapp, S. E. *et al.*: Thelaziasis in Cats and Dogs, J.A.V.M.A., *138*, 537, 1961.
14. Castroviejo, Ramon: Plastic and Reconstructive Surgery of the Conjunctiva, J. Plastic and Recons. Surgery, *24*, p. 9, 1959.
15. Spaeth, Edmund B.: *Principles and Practice of Ophthalmic Surgery*, 4th ed., Philadelphia, Lea & Febiger, p. 607, 1948.

Chapter 6

DISEASES AND SURGERY OF THE CORNEA AND SCLERA

Anatomy and Physiology

6:1   The cornea[1] is the clear, transparent, anterior segment of the external fibrous tunic of the eyeball. It is almost circular and, like the globe as a whole, it varies in dimensions between the breeds. The diameter will vary from 12.5 to 17 mm and there is seldom more than 1 mm difference in the vertical and horizontal meridional measurements. The vertical meridian has the smaller dimension. The radius of curvature is usually about 8 mm, but the radii of the anterior and posterior surfaces differ as the cornea is thicker in the center (0.73 to 0.95 mm) than at the periphery (0.6 to 0.8 mm). This is contrary to the form of the human cornea (0.6 mm thickness).

6:2   The cornea in the dog has but *four* distinct layers (Fig. 73): *epi-*

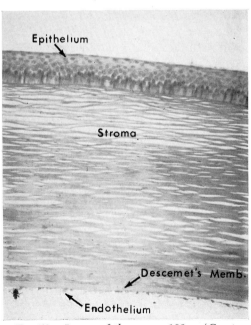

Fig. 73.   Layers of the cornea 100×. (Courtesy of Dr. A. C. Andersen, Davis, Cal.)

87

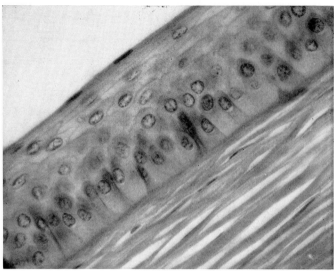

Fig. 74.   Corneal epithelium 450×. (Courtesy of Dr. A. C. Andersen, Davis, Cal.)

thelium (0.08 mm thick); *stroma* (substantia propria) (0.5 to 0.6 mm thick); *Descemet's* membrane, which is about four times the thickness of the endothelium; and, *endothelium,* which is just one row of cells. Oda and Fukuda[2] were unable to recognize Bowman's membrane (as in man) by electron microscopic studies of the canine cornea.

6:3   The *epithelium* has its basal layer of columnar cells surmounted by from two to four layers of polyhedral and four to ten layers of squamous cells (Fig. 74). Practically it can be considered a *continuation* of the *bulbar conjunctiva.*

6:4   The *stroma,* comprising 90 per cent of the corneal thickness, consists of connective tissue arranged in lamellae which are broad bands of interlacing collagenous fibrils extending over the entire width of the cornea and arranged parallel to its surface. Fixed corneal cells (corpuscles) lie in the lamellar interspaces where they are flattened and compressed. Leukocytes (wandering cells) are found in the lamellar inter-

spaces. A rich nerve supply enters the middle layer of the stroma, runs forward in a radial fashion to the center of the cornea and terminates as a plexus under the epithelium, with free nerve endings running between the epithelial cells.[3] The stroma of the cornea *passes* uninterruptedly *into* the *sclera.*

6:5   *Descemet's membrane* is a thin, firm, structureless, transparent, and highly *elastic* layer which often remains when all other layers are destroyed, and then gives rise to a descemetocele (Par. 6:112).

6:6   The *endothelium* consists of a single layer of cells (4 μ thick) lying over the inner surface of Descemet's membrane. Both of these layers are *continuous* with the *iris* and *ciliary* body.

6:7   The transition area between the cornea and the conjunctiva and sclera is known as the *limbus* (Par. 1:16). The area is rich in blood vessels and nerve endings and is marked by an oblique line of pigment cells which may, in some normal eyes, extend between the corneal lamellae for some distance beyond the corneoscleral junction.

Physiology

6:8   The cornea is an avascular tissue, receiving its nutrition through a process of dialysis from the perilimbal vessel plexus (Fig. 75) and, to a lesser extent, from the aqueous and tears.

6:9   The cornea consists largely of protein, namely, mucoid, collagen, elastin, albumin and globulin. Collagen is present in the greatest concentration and is one of the factors involved in wound healing. A delay in its formation has been demonstrated in vitamin C deficiency. I have administered, on occasions, vitamin C intravenously to dogs, in which an ulcerous area of the cornea had failed to heal, with a dramatic response and rapid regeneration.

6:10   The corneal proteins play an important part in acid burns of the cornea. When acid touches the cornea, its proteins are immediately precipitated by the acid. This precipitate in turn acts as a barrier to the further penetration of the acid into the deeper structures of the cornea (Fig. 76). This phenomenon, then, accounts for the fact that it is possible to use carbolic acid and trichloracetic acid for cauterizing purposes without danger of perforation. In contrast, alkalies do not form a precipitate with the proteins of the cornea,

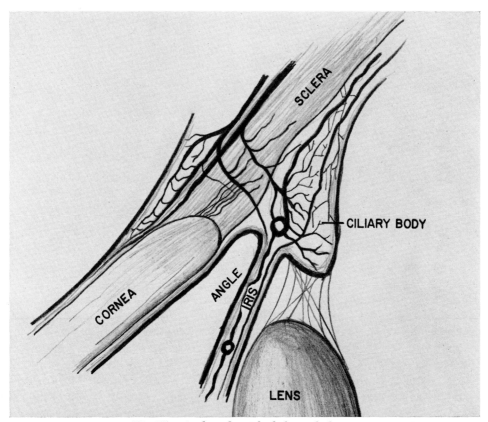

Fig. 75.   Angle and peri-limbal vessel plexus.

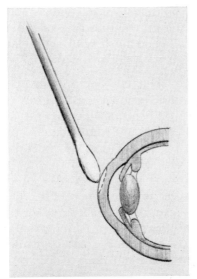

Fig. 76. Acid application to cornea with resultant precipitate (dotted line) barring further acid penetration.

but rather pass through and in many instances cause irreparable damage.

6:11   Most of the corneal metabolism is carried out by the epithelium. Other dietary deficiencies influencing this metabolism include riboflavin, a lack of which will result in vascularization of the cornea. Vitamin A, while more important to the well-being of the retina, is known to have a definite influence on epithelial cells and so may well be of importance also in the metabolism of the cornea.

6:12   The endothelium and epithelium control of the water content of the cornea. Since it is well established that the corneal stroma has a marked affinity for water, it is important that an intact epithelium and endothelium be maintained. Otherwise, edema and loss of transparency result. The endothelium is more important than the epithelium in this respect, since it is possible to lose considerable epithelium without showing corneal edema, but

minimal loss of endothelium, if it is not regenerated immediately, results in demonstrable corneal edema (opacity) This has been demonstrated often in instances of epithelial ulceration, with little or no accompanying edema, versus the severe edema, with resultant opacity, that accompanies injury to the endothelium through disease (Par. 7:32), or following intraocular surgery.

6:13   The transparency of the cornea also becomes temporarily impaired when abnormal pressures are applied to it With the sudden rise of intraocular pressure in acute glaucoma, the cornea becomes cloudy (Par. 9:20). Once this pressure is relieved, the cloudiness disappears.

6:14   To maintain the transparency of the cornea it must be bathed with a fluid having an osmotic pressure higher than interstitial fluid. If the cornea is bathed with a hypotonic solution, it becomes cloudy due to the loss of the osmotic forces acting on the corneal epithelium. When the cornea is cloudy because it is edematous, it can be cleared temporarily by bathing the eye with a hypertonic solution, such as 10 per cent salt or glycerin solution. Often it is necessary to do this in order to proceed with ophthalmoscopy or to view the iris and lens.

6:15   The cornea is an extremely sensitive structure, being richly supplied with free nerve endings (Par. 6:4). An insensitive cornea, in which a reflex is absent while being "feathered" with a wisp of cotton, is a prominent diagnostic sign of glaucoma in the dog (Par. 9:22). It also has been noted frequently that in those corneal lesions accompanied by extreme photophobia and pain, the lesion is situated in the superficial layers of the cornea and the more severe the photophobia is, the more superficial the pathologic process is likely to be. An eye that does not appear to be involved in any way, except for the discomfort shown, will often take a fluorescein stain over a large but very superficial area. It is believed that the pain and photophobia is due largely to vasodilatation taking place in the ciliary body. Thus the use of atropine to dilate the pupil and paralyze the ciliary body will alleviate the pain and photophobia (Par. 3:27).

6:16 All of the layers of the cornea are capable of spontaneous regeneration, with the exception of Descemet's, which depends upon the endothelium for regeneration. Epithelial regeneration takes place by sliding or migration of cells, or by multiplication of cells (mitosis). The migratory activity occurs first and almost immediately following an abrasion of the cornea. Cell division follows shortly. It has been shown, however, that small epithelial defects may be healed entirely without any cell multiplication—simply by cell migration. The rapidity with which these changes occur often has been evident in dogs in which the cornea takes a stain immediately following an abrasion (denoting loss of epithelium), only to exhibit complete regeneration twenty-four hours later, when a second attempt at staining fails.

6:17 Almost anything used on the cornea will interfere with corneal regeneration. The least of all would be saline solution. Ointments retard more than solutions of drugs, with the exception of local anesthetics, in which the reverse is true. Powders are still more deleterious in their effect on regeneration. With this information in mind, the careful clinician will then use drugs on the abrasions or ulcers of the cornea only as long as it is necessary to bring a possible infection under control. Anesthetic agents should be used sparingly, if at all, in the daily treatment. Many a stubborn, non-healing ulcer has healed quickly, following cessation of all medication to the eye.

Congenital Anomalies of the Cornea

6:18 *Dermoid.* (Plate 4A) This embryological defect, in which a piece of skin tissue carries hair roots, may involve the cornea alone or both the conjunctiva and cornea (Par. 5:17). The anomaly is noticed by the owner soon after the lid separation takes place.

6:19 Often there are no associated symptoms or corneal lesions noted until the hair follicles in the dermoid grow longer. If irritative symptoms should occur before the puppy reaches an age where an anesthetic can be safely administered and the eye approached surgically, instillation of castor oil or cod liver oil will lubricate and protect the cornea. A superficial keratectomy (Par. 6:152) with complete excision of the dermoid (Fig. 77A and B) is usually performed at about three months of age. The use of an antibiotic ointment for several days following surgery is sufficient. The cornea regenerates rapidly and usually without a trace of a scar.

6:20 *Microcornea* is usually associated with microphthalmos (Par. 8:12), a not uncommon hereditary anomaly in the poodle, miniature schnauzer and collie breeds.

6:21 *Megalophthalmos* (hydrophthalmos, buphthalmia) results from developmental defects of the filtration area of the chamber angle. The extensible sclera and cornea of the puppy is unable to withstand the raised tension

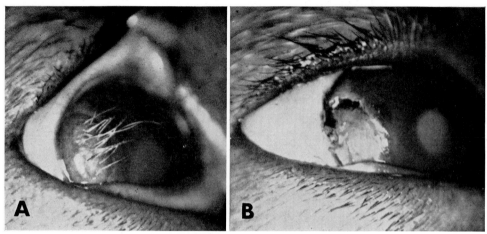

Fig. 77.   A. Corneal dermoid. B. Immediately following removal.

and the whole globe becomes enlarged. I have observed this condition (congenital glaucoma) but once, in a cocker spaniel puppy.

Keratitis[5]
Characteristics of Keratitis

6:22   Inflammation of the cornea generally presents one or more of the following objective signs: (1) loss of transparency, (2) ciliary injection, (3) vascularization, (4) cellular deposits in the aqueous, and (5) ulceration.

6:23   (1) *Loss of transparency* may be partial or complete and may result from (*a*) a change in the water content of the cornea (edema) (Par. 6:12); (*b*) increased intraocular pressure (glaucoma) (Par. 9:20); or (*c*) from an inflammatory exudate of one type or another, usually a leukocyte infiltration (Par. 7:32).

6:24   (2) *Ciliary injection* (Par. 5:16). The circumcorneal vessels, which are derived from the anterior ciliary vessels, become engorged in varying degrees. The conjunctival vessels often appear injected too, especially if the keratitis is an extension of a conjunctivitis.

6:25   (3) *Vascularization.*[6] Since the cornea is an avascular tissue, (Par. 6:8), in order to increase its defenses against irritants in pathological conditions, metabolism is increased; first, by an augmentation of the normal circulation, which is evident clinically as a pericorneal injection; and secondly, by the actual invasion of the cornea itself by

Plate 4.

A. Dermoid cyst involving conjunctiva and cornea.
B. Corneal dystrophy.
C. Superficial vascularization of the cornea. Note extension from the bulbar conjunctiva.
D. Interstitial (deep) keratitis. Note "brush-like" invasion of the vessels and the opacity resulting from the severe corneal edema.
E. Pannus of the German Shepherd. Right eye. Note invasion from the lateral limbal area.
F. Atypical inflammatory pannus. Note "cobblestone" cornea and swollen membrane nictitans.
G. Exuberant granulation tissue. Note large trunk vessels supplying the area.
H. Pigmentary keratitis. Note conjunctival melanin invasion onto the cornea.

Plate 4

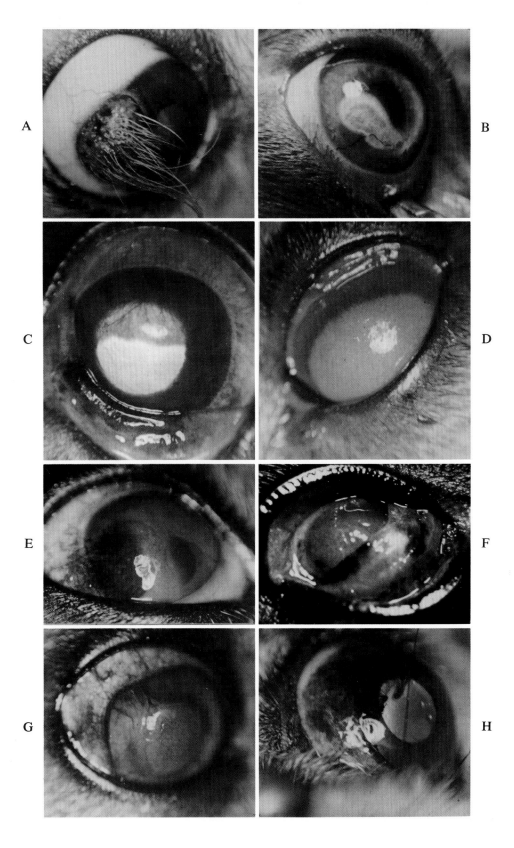

new vessels. Pericorneal injection is the invariable accompaniment of inflammatory or irritative precesses in the cornea, and is, essentially, the engorgement of the normal perilimbal plexus, which is usually microscopically invisible.

6:26 Adler[7] concludes that most diseases of the cornea result in its vascularization, and the type of vessels and their location in the cornea are often clues to the nature of the disease process. The diseases which commonly affect *epithelial structures* are accompanied by *superficial vascularization*, the vessels coming across the limbus from the conjunctiva. Those diseases affecting *parenchymatous tissues*, on the other hand, are characterized by *deep vessels*, coming from the anastomosis of the long posterior ciliary arteries and the anterior ciliary arteries. Once the cornea has become vascularized, the vessels remain throughout life. They are frequently empty of blood (ghost vessels), but their presence can always be detected with suitable magnification, and are testimony to the fact that the cornea has been the seat of a previous inflammatory process.

6:27 Once the process of vascularization is understood a more accurate prognosis and the proper choice of treatment can be determined. The two types of vascularization are referred to as *superficial* and *deep*, and from their appearance in the cornea are easily distinguishable one from the other (Plate 4C and D).

6:28 The superficial vessels run directly under the epithelium and in the superficial stroma and can often be seen as a continuation of vessels in the adjacent bulbar conjunctiva. They are a bright red and branch in tree-like fashion.

6:29 The deep vessels, since they are derived from the deep ciliary vessels, disappear from view at the margin of the cornea as they run into the sclera. They are a darker purple color and appear as long straight lines or form brush-like clumps.

6:30 (4) *Cellular deposits in the aqueous*, often referred to as "aqueous flare," is an indication that the neighboring deep parts (iris and ciliary body) are also involved. The turbidity may be slight, or a hypopyon (pus in the anterior chamber) may develop. The pus is an exudation from the iris and ciliary body when these parts participate in the inflammation (Par. 7:32).

6:31 (5) *Ulceration* may be superficial or deep, spreading or stationary. The extent of ulceration is best detected by the use of fluorescein (Par. 3:68) which stains green all ulcerated or abraded parts. Aside from the loss of corneal substance there is nearly always some grayish infiltration immediately surrounding the ulceration.

6:32 *Subjective* symptoms of keratitis include pain, photophobia, lacrimation, and blepharospasm. These symptoms may be slight or pronounced, depending upon the type of keratitis.

Classification of Keratitis

6:33 Diseases of the cornea have been variously classified under the etiology, topical and histologic localization, and clinical and pathologic features of their early or late manifestations. It will always be difficult to type or classify every case of keratitis. Overlapping or concurrent findings tend to obscure the picture. For the sake of simplicity and to render a discussion of therapeutic measures more realistic, the following classification, based on the most salient features presented at the time, is suggested.

- A. Superficial keratitis
  1. Superficial punctate keratitis
  2. Superficial dystrophies
  3. Superficial vascularization
  4. Pannus
  5. Exuberant granulation tissue
  6. Bullous keratitis
  7. Keratitis sicca
- B. Pigmentary keratitis
- C. Deep (Interstitial) keratitis
- D. Ulcerative keratitis
  1. Simple
  2. Deep
  3. Serpent or dendritic
  4. Nutritional
  5. Corneal erosion

A. Superficial Keratitis

6:34 A general diagnosis of superficial keratitis is made when the involvement is limited to the epithelium and superficial part of the stroma, and when there is no true ulceration.

6:35 *1. Superficial punctate keratitis*

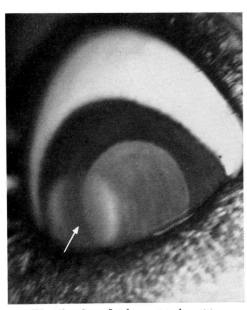

Fig. 78. Superficial punctate keratitis.

(Fig. 78) is characterized by the presence of epithelial and subepithelial opacities or infiltrates which do not take a stain. With magnification they appear as tiny white dots which give the involved portion of the cornea a stippled appearance. The condition is spontaneous in nature, and there is no accompanying corneal or conjunctival pathology. It is most often limited to the central part of the cornea.

6:36 *Etiology.* There would appear to be no one cause for the appearance of this type lesion in the cornea. External influences, *i.e.* wind and dust, may be a factor. A localized virus could possibly be incriminated as it is in a similar corneal lesion of man.

6:37 *Treatment.* The condition appears to be self-limiting, since usually the punctate opacities leave the cornea within several months to a year and do not return. Yellow mercuric oxide (2 per cent) ointment (Par. 3:18) seems to be of help in the dissipation of the lesion through its abrasive action. It is prescribed for use twice a day over a period of not to exceed two months. On occasion the tiny discrete opacities not only fail to leave the cornea, but coalesce, become denser, and result in a type of corneal dystrophy (Par. 6:38). In these instances it is necessary to resort to surgical removal of the involved epithelium and superficial stroma (Par. 6:152), or simply ignore the lesion unless vision is interfered with.

6:38 *2. Superficial dystrophies* (Fig. 79A, B and C) (Plate 4B) embrace an obscure category of superficial degenerative corneal lesions in the dog. The classification is used only for lack of a better one at present. The condition is slowly progressive, non-inflammatory, and, usually unilateral. The area of in-

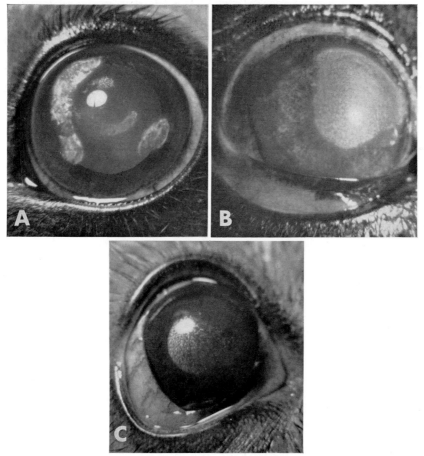

Fig. 79. Corneal dystrophies.

volvement has a granular, glistening, ground glass appearance. In time, several blood vessels will be noted extending from the limbus to the lesion in an effort to repair the damage. Melanin deposition may follow (Par. 6:64).

6:39 *Etiology.* Some cases may follow an ocular inflammatory disease, but, for the majority, no cause can be elicited.

6:40 *Treatment.* A superficial keratectomy (Par. 6:152) is indicated in those instances in which the lesion is progressing, becomes disfiguring, or interfers with vision. Regeneration of normal stromal and epithelial tissue takes place following surgery and the cornea remains perfectly clear. On occasion, in cases of long standing, the dystrophy will have invaded the deeper stroma. In these instances some haze may remain following regeneration of the overlying tissue.

6:41 3. *Superficial vascularization* of the cornea may occur as the result of:

a. Injury, *e.g.*, foreign bodies in the cornea, distichiasis, or neoplasms of the lid rubbing on the cornea. Following removal of the exciting cause, the cornea clears without need for further treatment.

b. Infection. An extension of a purulent conjunctivitis (keratoconjunctivitis) will provoke superficial vascularization. Control of the infection with the proper antibiotic-steroid combination will, in turn, result in clearing.

c. Allergy. Sensitivity to allergens, *e.g.* pollens, will produce a transient vessel invasion. Also included in this classification are those obscure cases of so-called atypical pannus in which there is some corneal opacity and melanin deposition accompanying the superficial vascularization. Topical steroid or antihistamine steroid therapy is specific, but treatment must be continued so long as the eyes are exposed to whatever the allergen might be.

d. Nutritional. Diet deficiencies, especially a lack of riboflavin, may result in superficial vascularization. The cornea clears quickly following correction of the diet and the administration of riboflavin (15 mg daily). Vascularization produced by nutritional deficiency is uncommon today but its possibility must be considered when no other cause can be determined.

6:42   4. *Pannus* (Plate 4E) is defined as a subepithelial connective-tissue infiltration of the cornea with accompanying vascularization.[8, 9] There is a particular predisposition to this disease in the German shepherd breed. Numerous sections removed and submitted by me to the Armed Forces Institute of Pathology (Ophthalmic Registry) have been given this designation (Pannus) (Fig. 80). Other authors have described this lesion in the German shepherd and have variously classified it as chronic superficial keratitis, pterygium, pseudo-pterygium or corneal metaplasia.

6:43   The lesion begins as a grayish haze at the limbus. In most instances it affects both eyes and begins on the temporal side (9:00 o'clock position on the right eye; 3:00 o'clock on the left eye). The film, with accompanying blood vessels and pigment, continues to spread over the cornea until it is eventually covered, with blindness resulting. With the aid of biomicroscopy (Par. 2:6) white infiltrates and "peppery" melanin deposits can be seen preceding the grossly observable lesion into what appears to be clear corneal tissue.

6:44   The disease takes several forms. The spread on the cornea may be slow and otherwise symptom free, or, it may assume a very inflammatory form in which a rapid "cobblestone" build-up is noted on the cornea and in which the conjunctiva, including the membrane nictitans, is obviously a part of the inflammation (Plate 4F). An accompanying catarrhal discharge can be expected in this form.

6:45   *Etiology.* The cause is unknown. Überreiter[10] was unable to incriminate a bacterial component or effect an innoculation in healthy controls. I have been unsuccessful also in this attempt. Environmental conditions do not seem to be of importance because the disease is encountered throughout the United States and many parts of the world in those dogs confined to the home as well as those in a constant outside exposure.

6:46   *Treatment.* Until a cause is determined, the treatment of pannus will remain frustrating. Destruction or removal of the lesion is simple enough, but constant steroid therapy is necessary in most cases to prevent return of the lesion. Lamellar corneal grafts to replace removed diseased tissue, and the use of autologous or homologous conjunctival grafts have been used in an unsuccessful attempt to prevent return of the lesion. X-ray and beta-ray irradiation have been given a thorough trial and found to be wanting. Early pannus often responds well to irradiation initially, only to recur. Small repeated doses and single massive doses of beta-ray irradiation have been tried and the results do not differ appreciably, with a temporary remission only resulting.

6:47 Steroid therapy, employing the subconjunctival method (Par. 3:56) is the preferred treatment in early pannus and is *especially* valuable in the inflammatory type mentioned (Par. 6:44). Three or so injections at forty-eight-hour intervals will cause regression of the lesion and clearing of the cornea of all but some residual haze and pigment. Concurrent and follow-up instillation of steroid-antibiotic combinations in drop or ointment form twice a day will ordinarily prevent a relapse and return of the pathology to these hypersensitive eyes. Long continued use of the steroids may lead to fungal growth and corneal ulceration (Par. 6:86). If and when this complication occurs the steroid therapy is discontinued until the reparative process is complete. A steroid-antibiotic-fungicidal preparation, Panolog,* is then used. An insidious invasion of the pannus may also take place in spite of this type therapy, thus requiring the additional procedures of either peritomy (Par. 6:51), chemical cautery with carbolic-acid, or a superficial keratectomy. Occasionally a patient responds well to a change of the steroid preparation. The reason for this remains obscure.

6:48 Pure carbolic-acid cauterization of a pannus area has proven to be

* Panolog. Squibb, New York, N. Y.

a more rapid and satisfactory means of destroying the metaplastic tissue than either x-ray or beta radiation. Cautery with phenol is most effective in the early stages before the "build-up" becomes too pronounced. A cotton applicator is impregnated with phenol by the drop method and then is rubbed over the affected portion of the cornea until the area is well blanched. A rinse with the standard eye wash (Par. 3:11) is all that is needed after the application. The diseased tissue will slough from the underlying stroma and regeneration will readily take place, but relapse and return of the pannus will occur later unless, as previously mentioned, steroid therapy is continued.

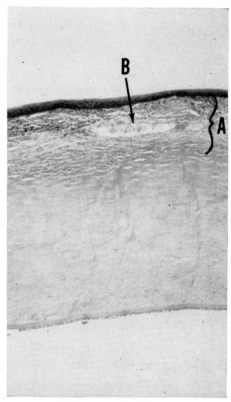

Fig. 80. Photomicrograph of pannus. *A,* area of infiltration; *B,* blood vessel.

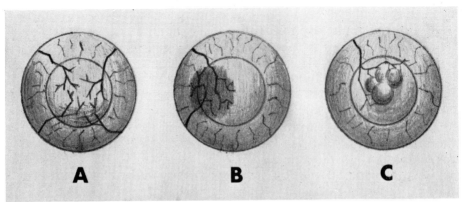

Fig. 81. *A.* Superficial vascularization (vessels only). *B.* Pannus. Subepithelial connective tissue infiltration accompanied by superficial vascularization. *C.* Exuberant granulation tissue. Superficial vessels "feeding" granulation.

6:49 Performing a superficial keratectomy provides the quickest and most effective way of ridding a cornea of the lesion. Ordinarily, however, this procedure is reserved for those eyes in which the greater part of the cornea is involved or when it offers the only hope of restoring vision. The technique is described under Surgical Procedures (Par. 6:152). Following the keratectomy the underlying stroma will be found to be crystal clear and a blind animal will have vision restored immediately (Fig. 116C). Following corneal regeneration the aforementioned steroid therapy is commenced.

6:50 5. *Exuberant granulation tissue* (Plate 4G) builds up on the cornea as the result of injury or ulceration. Superficial vessels can be seen extending from the conjunctiva, thence across the cornea to the area of granulation. Granulation tissue should not be confused with either true pannus or simple superficial vascularization (Fig. 81).

6:51 *Treatment.* By peritomy, using either heat or electrocautery, the source of blood supply to the granulation areas is destroyed at its origin where it arises in the bulbar conjunctiva (Fig. 82).

Without the support of these vessels, the granulation tissue will disappear, and the cornea will regain its transparency. Each vessel leading from the conjunctiva to the corneal granulation tissue is touched with the cautery just back of the limbus. A steroid preparation may be used afterwards to expedite the dissipation of the vessels and granulation tissue. *Caution*—so long as the ulcerous or abraded area stains, it is best to delay peritomy until the healing process is near complete.

6:52 6. *Bullous keratitis* (Plate 5A and Fig. 101). In bullous keratopathy tiny vacuoles in the epithelium coalesce to form vesicles and edema in the superficial corneal tissues. These vesicles are also known as bullae. The area involved becomes very edematous and opaque, whereas the surrounding cornea may be perfectly clear.

6:53 *Etiology.* The condition usually occurs as a result of injury or ulceration. In these particular instances there is an abnormal absorption of fluid through the break in the epithelium (Par. 6:12).

6:54 *Treatment* is symptomatic. The

bullae may be smoothed off with eye scissors and the eye treated open as an ulcerative keratitis (Par. 6:94). In severe cases the use of the membrane nictitans as a conjunctival flap is the preferred procedure (Par. 5:65). The prognosis is ordinarily good because of the superficial nature of the condition.

6:55 7. *Keratitis sicca* (dry cornea) is characterized by discomfort and *photophobia* of one or both eyes and a loss of the usual glistening appearance of the cornea. The disease is caused by an insufficiency of lacrimal secretion. The lacrimal gland fails to produce tears and the accessary glands no longer produce the viscid precorneal film which is so important to the well being of the cornea (Par. 4:4).

6:56 The conjunctiva becomes red, thickened, and velvety (Par. 5:46), a sticky, ropy secretion invariably accompanies the condition. These findings often leads the clinician wrongly to assume that a chronic bacterial conjunctivitis is responsible. Upon staining, however, it will be noted that the cornea takes a very light stain over its entire surface. This is most evident when viewed with suitable magnification. A *dry nostril* on the affected side offers further evidence that the lacrimal secretion is insufficient. The lacrimal drainage apparatus is usually patent but is simply non-functional because of the lack of secretion.

6:57 *Etiology.* The causes for cessation of or insufficient lacrimal secretion are varied and include the following: (*a*) *chronic distemper*. Upon full recovery from the systemic disease the lacrimal function returns with a resultant clearing of the discharge and return of corneal luster. (*b*) *Injuries* to the head may result in atrophy of the secreting glands and surrounding musculature with but little hope for return of function. (*c*) A chronic *blepharitis/conjunctivitis* syndrome may, in turn, affect the function of the glands either temporarily or permanently. (*d*) *Senility* in itself may be a factor. (*e*) *Congenital*

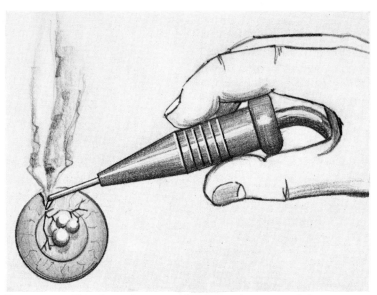

Fig. 82.   Destruction of blood supply to granulation area by means of electrocautery peritomy.

absence of or malfunction of the secreting glands has been encountered in several breeds (Yorkshire terriers, chihauhaus, miniature pinchers).

6:58   *Treatment.* Artificial tear therapy (Par. 3:90) with or without the addition of antibiotics must be continued until the secreting function returns, as in the case of distemper, or, indefinitely in those conditions mentioned in which permanent loss of function is evident. Commerical preparations of artificial tears (methyl-cellulose solution) are available under different trade names. *Parralog*

B. *Pigmentary Keratitis*

6:59   A special classification is accorded so-called pigmentary keratitis (keratitis pigmentosa) because of its prevalence. Actually, the condition as such does qualify under the heading of superficial keratitis since usually only this portion of the cornea is involved. Neither should pigmentary keratitis be thought of as a disease entity in itself since it almost invariably is *secondary* to another disease process.

6:60   Roberts' study[11] indicates that practically all pigment in the cornea is melanin and that pigmentation of the superficial cornea originates in the germinal epithelium and, to a limited extent, from the limbus (Par. 6:7). The germinal epithelium has the same embryological origin as that of the conjunctiva, where pigment is found naturally (Par. 5:4).

6:61   Michaelson[12] conducted experiments which are important to the understanding of pigmentary keratitis in the dog. He found that when an artificial lesion is made in the cornea of the rabbit, there is, besides an intrusion of the new blood vessels from the limbus, a proliferation or "sliding" of the conjunctival epithelial cells *including* pigment cells into the cornea. This report indicates that proliferation of the limbal melanoblasts into the cornea is apparently, under certain circumstances, a constant reaction to an experimental lesion of the cornea in the rabbit, that the proliferation has certain features in common with the vascular proliferation and occurs at the same time, and that both proliferations are probably due to the same stimulus. As pointed out earlier (Par. 6:7), the limbal area of the dog is similarly marked by a line of pigment.

6:62   *Etiology.* There are four possible reasons for the deposition of melanin in the cornea.

6:63   1. *Stress.* Melanin from the bulbar conjunctiva and limbal area enters the cornea in the presence of a stress factor. Distichiasis (Par. 4:30) ranks as a primary exciting factor. The rubbing of lashes on the bulbar conjunctiva and cornea of the protruding eye, especially in the pekingese and pug breeds, causes the migration of the pigment onto the cornea (Plate 4H). Long hairs arising from the prominent nasal folds are also a direct cause for pigment deposition in the medial aspect of the cornea. Entropion, chronic purulent conjunctivitis, keratitis sicea, and pannus also predispose to the migration of the pigment.

6:64   2. *Following and accompanying superficial vascularization,* as noted also by Roberts[11] and Michaelson.[12] Actually, vascularization, whether it be deep or superficial, is also the result of an exciting stress factor (inflammation), which in turn results in the migration of pigment.

6:65   3. *As a sequela to deep (inter-*

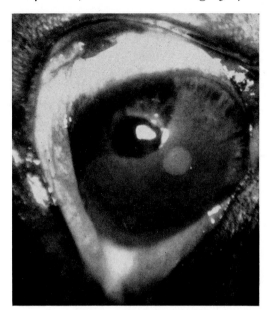

Fig. 83. Pigmentary keratitis as a sequel to interstitial keratitis.

stitial) keratitis (Fig. 83). When interstitial keratitis (Par. 6:82) is not recognized as such and is allowed to run its course without the proper treatment, there is often a residual pigment deposition. This, in most instances, is melanin, but hemosiderin deposition resulting from a breakdown of blood vessels in the cornea also may be a contributing factor.

6:66   4. *Migration of uveal pigment* (Fig. 84). Following corneal perforation and iris prolapse, an anterior synechia between iris and cornea often results. It is then that uveal pigment migrates through and along the natural nerve and vessel openings and deposits itself in the corneal stroma and on the surface.

6:67   *Treatment.* Since stress or an exciting factor of some sort is always responsible for the presence of corneal pigment, the first consideration is to determine and eliminate the cause. It is somewhat incongruous to persist in

the removal of the unwanted pigment only to see its return because of a failure to recognize the cause for its presence.

6:68   If distichiasis or trichiasis is the exciting factor, the lashes must be removed (Par. 4:33). Long hairs arising from prominent nasal folds must, of course, be kept trimmed to prevent their reaching the cornea. Better still, surgical removal of the redundant folds offers a more satisfactory and permanent method of eliminating this source of irritation. As a bonus, this procedure is also of benefit in those instances in which there is an accompanying chafing dermatitis.

6:69   The surgical procedure is performed simply by preparing the site through close clipping and the usual skin preparation (Fig. 85A). The exposed ridges are excised at their bases, flush with the surrounding skin, with heavy surgical scissors. The incisions will ordinarily meet above the nose as an inverted V. Interrupted or mattress

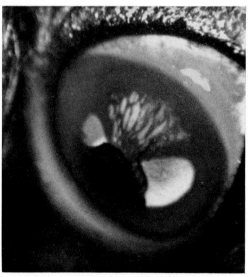

Fig. 84.   Migration of uveal pigment with deposition on the cornea.

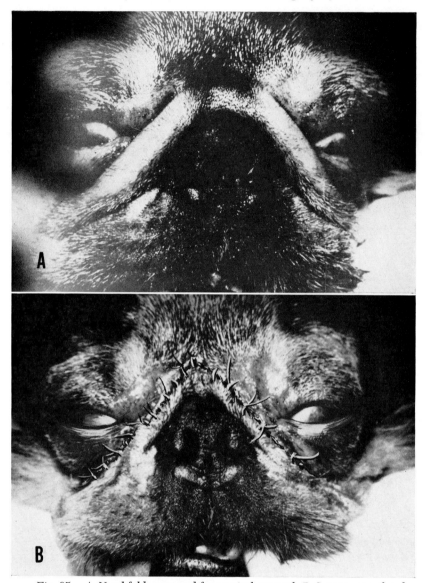

Fig. 85.   A. Nasal folds prepared for surgical removal. B. Surgery completed.

sutures complete the procedure (Fig. 85B).

6:70   Surgical correction of entropion (Par. 4:20) is necessary to prevent further excitation of pigment from that cause. In cases of chronic purulent conjunctivitis (Par. 5:40), the pigment migration cannot be controlled until all inflammation and discharge is cleared from the eye. Elimination of pannus (Par. 6:42) and prevention of its return by one of the means previously described are also essential to the control of the accompanying pigmentation.

6:71   It can be quite definitely stated that proper and prompt handling of interstitial keratitis is the best deterrent to the type of pigmentary keratitis which often follows.

6:72 Following the elimination of the exciting cause, little attention need be paid the pigment unless the pupillary area is occluded and vision impaired. If it is necessary that the pigment be removed, this is easily performed by either scraping it from the cornea with, for example, a No. 15 blade (Fig. 86A), or sloughing it off with phenol cauterization (Fig. 86B). Peritomy (Par. 6:51, Fig. 82) of any accompanying trunk vessels on the conjunctival side may also be indicated.

6:73 Radiation in itself has been given a thorough trial[13] and found to be helpful, but also lacking in many respects. Essentially, radiation therapy is just another destructive device which, through its latent action, causes dissipation of pigment. This same objective can be attained far more readily by scraping and/or cautery.

6:74 Following removal of the pigment and the associated superficial layers, the eye is treated as though an ulcerative keratitis were present. Atropine drops for alleviation of pain, topical antibiotics to prevent infection, and vitamin therapy (Par. 3:64) to enhance regeneration of corneal epithelium is

used for the first five or six days. Thereafter, a steroid-antibiotic preparation is used to effect clearing.

6:75 Again, unless the pigment is interfering with vision, or needs to be removed for other reasons, it is best left alone. Uveal pigment deposited in and on the cornea should never be attacked surgically since it is possible to disrupt the "patch" between iris and cornea, and thereby produce a leaking anterior chamber or lost eye.

C. Deep (Interstitial) Keratitis

6:76 Interstitial keratitis is characterized by deep vascularization and opacity throughout the layers of the cornea (Plate 4D). The condition is an *indication of deep seated trouble*, with diffuse cellular infiltration and edema allied with inflammation of the iris and ciliary body (uveal tract). The cellular infiltration may be so extensive that the entire cornea has a diffusely opaque appearance like ground glass. Vascularization may be scant or so intense that the cornea has a reddish appearance. The deep short vessels radiate evenly from the limbus toward the center and may escape detection in the early stage

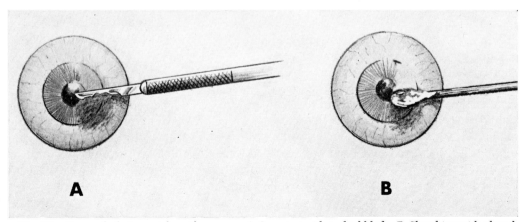

Fig. 86.   Removal of pigment from the cornea. A. Scraping with scalpel blade. B. Sloughing with phenol impregnated applicator.

of the disease. Later they become more prominent and progress in a brush-like pattern toward the center, but do not always reach to the center. The vascularization may confine itself to segments, but more often involves the whole circumference of the cornea. Occasionally a few superficial vessels will be noted extending over the limbus from the swollen conjunctiva toward the center of the cornea.

6:77 Because of the dense corneal opacity, often the iris cannot be seen and studied. In these instances it must be assumed that the keratitis is merely a part of a uveitis, participation of the uveal tract being hidden during the stage of opaque cornea.

6:78 *Etiology.* Causes of interstitial keratitis include: (1) focal infections, *e.g.*, tonsils, teeth, prostate, sinuses, endogenous toxin; (2) specific diseases, *e.g.*, distemper, hepatitis, toxoplasmosis; (3) wounds or ocular surgery; and (4) severe ulcerative keratitis. Any possible cause for the underlying uveitis must be considered. It is often difficult, if not impossible, to determine the exact cause, and considerable time must be spent in taking history, in a general physical examination, and in utilization of laboratory procedures.

6:79 *Treatment.* Since the appearance of the cornea and the type of vascularization denotes involvement of the uveal tract, treatment must be directed toward that structure. Again, the cause should first be determined and treated as such, if possible. If some systemic infection is found to be or even believed to be responsible, it is well to consider the systemic administration of chloromycetin (Par. 3:44) and/or the sulfonamides (Par. 3:46). Heat (Par. 3:71) in the form of hot moist compresses to the closed lids decreases pain and improves the circulation of the eye. Subconjunctival steroid injections (Par. 3:56) are most helpful in alleviating the corneal opacity (edema). Because of the posterior segment involvement, systemic steroids (Par. 3:56) often must also be used to achieve the best results. Foreign protein injections (Par. 3:69) may be of value but the steroids have largely supplanted their use.

6:80 X-ray radiation is of value for its palliative effect and for the discouragement of vascularization,[14] but is no longer important to the treatment of the disease since the advent of the steroids.

6:81 Paracentesis (Par. 6:143) would never be contraindicated and may well prove as effectual as it is in the treatment of uveitis (Par. 7:46).

6:82 *Complications and Sequelae.* In the event proper treatment has not been instigated or has been delayed, a secondary glaucoma sometimes occurs as a result of the uveitis (adhesions). Some corneal haze and deep corneal vessels may remain permanently. Often this is only discernible with good magnification. In chronic cases the cornea may become so softened by the infiltration that it bulges forward (ectasia) (Par. 6:119). Pigmentation of the cornea as a sequela has been discussed (Par. 6:65).

Endothelial Dystrophy

6:83 As opposed to epithelial dystrophy (Par. 6:38) in which only the superficial structures are involved, endothelial dystrophy produces a diffuse corneal involvement and thus is classified as a form of deep keratitis. The disease is not common but because of the hopelessness of treatment, a correct diagnosis is important. Mesenchymal dystrophy is a corneal change not due to an inflammatory agent nor to an allergic reaction, but is due rather to aging of tissues. I have encountered the disease in older dogs and have always found it to be bilateral. The underlying cause is believed to be a disturbance of the mesenchyme, with loss of its ability to prevent passage of the aqueous fluid into the corneal stroma.

6:84 On external appearance the entire cornea appears dull and mildly opaque, but the anterior chamber and underlying iris and lens can be seen. With the aid of a slit-lamp (Par. 2:5) or good oblique illumination and magnification, the posterior portion of the cornea appears edematous or infiltrated with fine opacities. Cataracts have been noted in conjunction with this dystrophy. Treatment instituted in the hope of clearing the cornea will be found to be fruitless.

D. *Ulcerative Keratitis*

6:85 Ulceration is the most common corneal disease encountered. Ulcerative keratitis denotes loss of substance of the cornea with or without accompanying corneal edema. The extent and degree of involvement is best determined by the use of fluorescein dye (Par. 2:19). The subjective symptoms of pain, photophobia, lacrimation and blepharospasm may be slight or pronounced. The extent of the ulcerative process has no bearing on the symptoms (Par. 6:15).

6:86 *Etiology.* Causes of loss of corneal substance include: injury (with subsequent infection), bacterial, viral, or fungal growths, nutritional, and *unknown*. Catcott and Griesemer[15] conclude that ulcerative keratitis is readily produced only when infectious organisms are introduced into an abraded sur-

face. A marked pathogenicity of *Pseudomonas aeruginosa* for the canine cornea has been shown in their experiments. The incidence of corneal ulceration due to fungi has been increasing as a result of fungal overgrowth from long-term antibiotic-steroid therapy (Par. 6:47). *Candida* or *Aspergillus* are the usual findings.[16] In suspected cases appropriate diagnostic procedures, including attempts to demonstrate fungi by smears and cultures, should be employed. Material for such studies should be obtained by scraping the cornea, since simple swabbing may yield nothing even though the infection is obvious.[17]

6:87 As is true with so many diseases of the eye, breed and strain incidence is of significance. The prominent eyes of the Pekingese, Pug and Boston terrier breeds apparently predispose to injury and infection. Also, the eyes in these breeds are often less responsive to treatment. Smythe[18] appropriately states that "corneal insufficiency is undoubtedly hereditary in certain breeding strains and it is noticeable how frequently corneal ulceration appears in some kennels and how infrequently in others, even when the conditions of feeding and management are equal."

6:88 *Classification.* Corneal ulcers may be classified in many ways, but for descriptive purposes the following is offered.

6:89 1. *Simple ulcer.* In this type the lesion remains small and superficial, with no tendency to spread or perforate. A simple nick or abrasion may be responsible. In most instances epithelial regeneration is rapid and complete in a few days.

6:90 2. *Deep ulcer* (Plate 5B). The tendency is to involve the deeper layers and cause perforation. The progress of this type of ulceration is rapid insofar as depth is concerned, but there is little tendency to spread over the cornea. Symptoms are marked, a bacterial component is present, and the iris may be involved, with pus in the anterior chamber (hypopyon).

6:91   3. *Serpent or dendritic ulcer* (branching like a tree) (Plate 5C). Usually associated with a systemic virus infection in the dog. The tendency is for the ulceration to spread, branch, and involve the deeper layers.

6:92   4. *Nutritional ulcer* (Plate 5D). The term *keratomalacia* is used to denote corneal ulceration due to an avitaminosis A, which, in turn, is due to lack of ingestion of vitamin A or to lack of its absorption from the gastrointestinal tract and proper utilization by the body. The entire cornea is dull and lusterless (mildly edematous) and the ulcer, while superficial, may involve a large area. The lesion really results from an erosion since the cornea becomes soft and necrotic. The condition is not common to the dog, but it is important that the cause be recognized since there will be no response to other than vitamin A therapy.

6:93   5. *Corneal erosion* (Plate 5E). This term is used to describe an ulceration peculiar to the boxer breed. The lesion is small, superficial, has no tendency to spread, presents an overhanging border all around (fluorescein stain) and there is no associated conjunctival discharge, corneal opacity, or vascularization in the early stages. The ulcer may remain stationary for long periods of time, during which the animal exhibits marked irritative symptoms, pain and photophobia. The cause is unknown. No bacterial or viral component has been found. Relapses following healing are common. Often some weeks or months later a new area of the cornea becomes involved or the fellow eye may be afflicted.

6:94   *Treatment of Ulcerative Keratitis:* Treatment of ulceration in general should embody methods which are aimed at control of the infection or erosion and hastening of the repair processes. Elimination of a possible cause, of course, must always be considered. Any corneal friction, *e.g.*, entropion, distichiasis, foreign bodies, may be directly responsible for the ulceration.

6:95   Ulcerative keratitis cases often need to be hospitalized. If treated on an out-patient basis, it is important that a re-examination be made in not to exceed forty-eight hours. Re-staining will indicate the progress of healing.

6:96   Cauterization (Par. 3:20) of most ulcers is important to the sterilization of the area, thus paving the way for regeneration. Tincture of iodine offers a very efficient mode of disinfecting and cauterizing ulcers. A piece of cotton

---

Plate 5.
  A. Bullous keratitis. Note clear area of cornea still remaining.
  B. Deep ulcer (fluorescein stained), vascularization, and hypopyon.
  C. Serpentine type of ulceration (fluorescein stained).
  D. Keratomalacia. Note stained area and accompanying corneal edema.
  E. Corneal erosion (fluorescein stained).
  F. Detergent denudation of the cornea (fluorescein stained).
  G. Chronic, non-healing ulcerative keratitis with granulation and pigmentation.
  H. Leaking descemetocele (center cornea), and pigmentation.

Plate 5

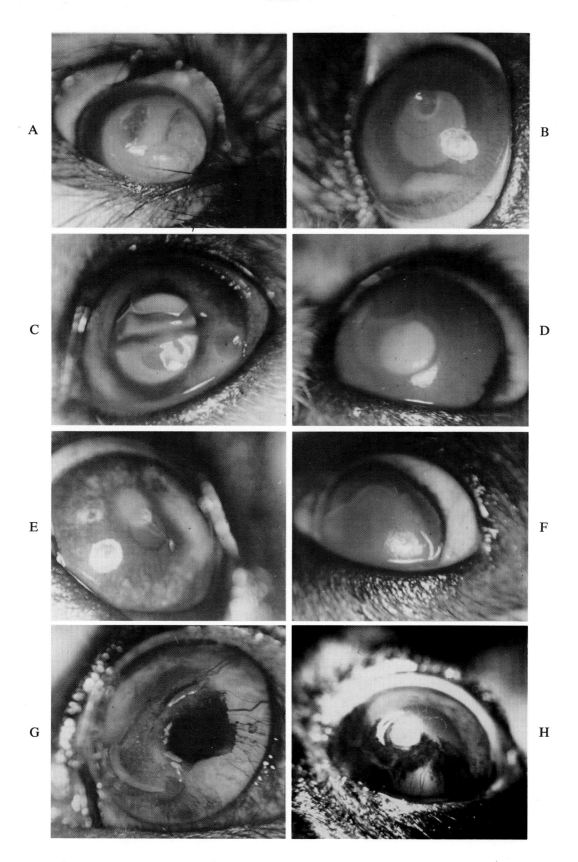

A

B

C

D

E

F

G

H

is wound tightly on the end of a tooth-pick, dipped into the iodine and then exposed to the air for a few seconds to rid the applicator of the excess. It is now brushed upon the ulcer, especially at its infiltrated margins (Fig. 87). This procedure can usally be accomplished under topical anesthesia. If the clinician feels that the ulcer needs further cauterization several days later, phenol may be used (Par. 3:22), although it is more destructive. Regardless of the type of cauterant used, the most important feature of the treatment is to cauterize an area 1 mm or more beyond the advancing margins of the ulcer.

6:97 Use of the antibiotic preparations (Par. 3:45) by topical instillation should be preceded by cleansing of the conjunctival sac (Par. 3:47). Systemic use of chloramphenicol (Par. 3:44) and/or chemotherapy (Par. 3:49) may be indicated in deep ulceration associated with hypopyon. The sodium succinate form of chloramphenicol has also been used by subconjunctival injection (Fig. 27) in this type of ulceration. Up to 75 mg may be injected in one area. Other antibiotics that may be administered by subconjunctival injection are: neomycin 10 to 100 mg; bacitracin 5,000 μ; and penicillin G crystalline 100,000 to 500,000 μ.

6:98 Non-specific protein therapy (Par. 3:67) is never contraindicated and is believed by many to be of value. Application of heat (Par. 3:71) is helpful, but its use is usually confined to the home. Enzymes (Par. 3:67) may be used systemically or orally as an aid to the absorption of hypopyon associated with deep ulceration.

6:99 Gamma globulin is presently undergoing investigative study in the treatment of ulceration. In man,[21] in-tramuscular injection with gamma globulin yielded favorable therapeutic results in 25 patients with various forms of viral keratitis. The course of the disease was shortened, subjective complaints mitigated, and the development of corneal scarring diminished or prevented. The use of gamma globulin by systemic administration and topical application has been tried in all types of ulceration in the dog but the results are, for the present, inconclusive. Subconjunctival injections of up to one-half cc appears to have promise in some ulcerative processes (Par. 6:107, 6:108).

6:100 Almost anything used on the cornea will have some effect on corneal regeneration (Par. 6:17). Thus, when an ulcerative process is well under control, consideration should be given to either stopping all medication or switching to preparations which will not interfere with final healing. The criteria for control includes: clearing of the discharges, filling in of the lesion (less staining), and relief from subjective symptoms.

6:101 Topical anesthetics have long been popular for affording pain relief in corneal injury or ulceration. Extensive research[19, 20] has established that

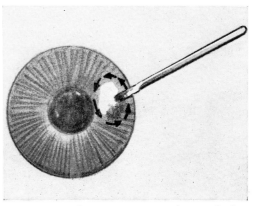

Fig. 87. Iodine cauterization of corneal ulcer using a cotton-wound toothpick.

topical application of most anesthetics inhibits mitosis in the intact epithelium, migration of epithelial cells over injured areas, and cell division in the regenerating epithelium. As mentioned (Par. 3:38), certain preparations may safely be used. Generally, however, an atropine instillation, once daily, will more adequately serve the purpose of relieving the discomfort associated with corneal abrasion or ulceration (Par. 3:27) and is to be preferred over the use of anesthetics.

6:102   The use of topical steroids is definitely contraindicated in abrasions or in corneal ulcers in which a bacterial or mycotic contamination is present or is apt to develop. Admittedly, steroids will decrease pain and minimize inflammatory response in corneal injuries, but this fosters a false sense of security. Sufficient evidence (Par. 3:51) has been gathered to emphasize the fact that many eyes have been lost because the detrimental effects of steroids were not appreciated. Steroids can be used, if needed, for relief of any associated inflammatory symptoms when healing is complete.

6:103   Hastening of the repair process is accomplished by the use of *vitamins* (Par. 3:63). *Bandaging* (Par. 3:80) is helpful, but only occasionally necessary. The use of a *conjunctival flap* (Par. 5:66) is one of the better means of promoting healing in chronic ulceration. *Paracentesis* (Par. 6:143) is indicated in deep ulceration, especially when a hypopyon is present.

6:104   A chronic, stagnant ulcerative process with accompanying vascularization, granulation, and pigmentation (Plate 5G) may need to be reversed by first sloughing off the top layers by *phenolization* (Par. 3:22). Or, a super-

ficial *keratectomy* (Par. 6:152) of the involved area may be necesary before the repair process can get off to a new, good start.

6:105   *Specific treatment* for the types of ulceration described varies with each case but, in general, the following may be applicable. (Please read the discussion of treatment in general before proceeding with specific therapy.)

6:106   1. *Simple ulcer*
    (*a*) Iodine cautery
    (*b*) Atropine
    (*c*) Topical antibiotic or vitamin A

6:107   2. *Deep ulcer*
    (*a*) Clean discharges
    (*b*) Iodine cautery (edges only)
    (*c*) Paracentesis
    (*d*) Atropine
    (*e*) Antibiotic therapy (topical, subconjunctival, systemic) and/or gamma globulin
    (*f*) Vitamins
    (*g*) Possible conjunctival flap

6:108   3. *Dendritic ulcer*
    (*a*) Clean discharges
    (*b*) Iodine cautery
    (*c*) Atropine
    (*d*) Antibiotics and/or gamma globulin
    (*e*) Vitamins
    (*f*) Possible conjunctival flap

6:109   4. *Nutritional ulcer*
    (*a*) Vitamin A
    (*b*) Topical treatment as needed

6:110   5. *Corneal erosion*
    A routine the author has

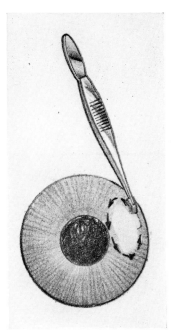

Fig. 88.   Stripping of overhanging epithelium in corneal erosion.

found helpful in the care of corneal erosion in the boxer is to, on admission:

(*a*) Strip the overhanging epithelium back several mm with eye tissue forceps (Fig. 88)

(*b*) Iodine cautery (Fig. 87)

(*c*) Atropine and a drop of **natural** vitamin A from a punctured 25,-000 unit capsule

(*d*) Intravenous ascorbic acid (500 mg) and niacin (100 mg)

The above can be accomplished under topical anesthesia, topical and/or tranquilizer, or short-acting barbiturate anesthesia. After care consists of: a drop of atropine daily, twice daily instillation of the vitamin A drops, and oral or injectable vitamins (Par. 3:63). Re-epithelialization is usually complete within five to seven days. Progress will first be evident when the irritative symptoms appear relieved. In instances where this treatment may fail to effect a cure, the use of a conjunctival flap must be considered.

Acquired Deformities of the Cornea (Fig. 89A, B, C, and D)

6:111   Protrusions or acquired deformities of the cornea may result from injury or ulcerative keratitis. They include: (1) descemetocele, (2) iris prolapse, (3) staphyloma, and (4) ectasia.

6:112   A *descemetocele* occurs when an ulceration proceeds down to Descemet's membrane (Fig. 90) and is warning that an iris prolapse is imminent.

6:113   *Treatment* includes paracentesis (Par. 6:144) and use of a conjunctival flap (Par. 5:65). Aftercare includes use of atropine and antibiotic instillations and vitamin therapy (Par. 3:64). Additional reinforcement can be achieved by bandaging (Par. 3:81). If bandaging is used, dressings are changed at forty-eight hour intervals. When the conjunctival flap is released after the usual one week period, good healing is noted and the danger of prolapse has passed. Roberts[22] advocates the use of lamellar corneal transplants as an aid to the repair of this lesion.

6:114   Occasionally the corneal defect, in association with a descemetocele or iris prolapse, will appear healed only to rupture some weeks or months later. Aqueous will escape and the anterior chamber will become shallow. Following this pressure relief, the wound will again seal with a filling of the chamber. This "weak patch" is thus subject to recurrent rupture and it is in these instances that a lamellar or penetrating keratoplasty procedure may be neces-

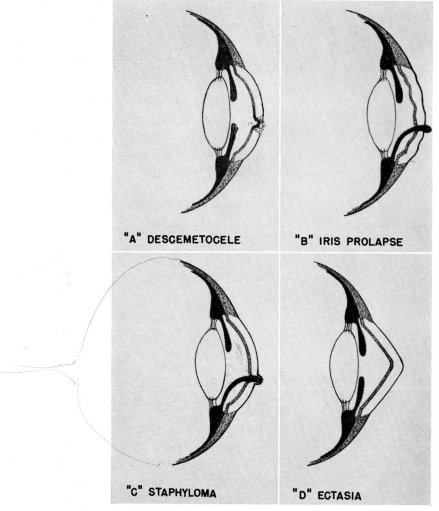

Fig. 89.   Acquired deformities of the cornea.
A. Descemetocele. B. Iris prolapse. C. Staphyloma. D. Ectasia.

Plate 6.

A. Iris prolapse.

B. Foreign body granuloma (result of embedded splinter).

C. Spongy granulomatous lesion of the episclera and cornea.

D. Nodular episcleritis (lower aspect of globe). Note accompanying corneal infiltration of vessels and pigment.

E. Inflammatory hyperplasia involving the conjunctiva and episclera.

F. Granuloma involving the episclera (side view). Note infiltration of the cornea.

G. Intrascleral invasion of a malignant melanoma of the uveal tract.

H. Malignant lymphoma. Note intraocular growth and corneal-scleral involvement.

Plate 6

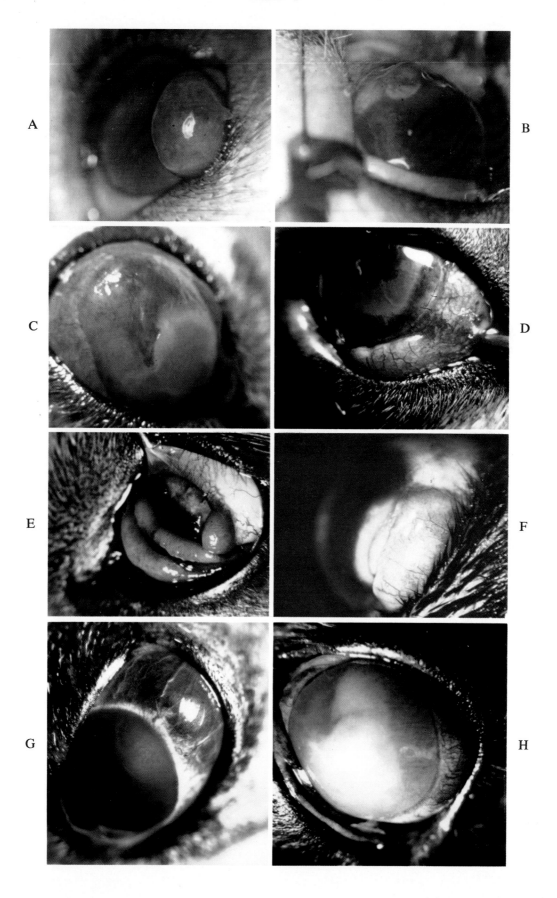

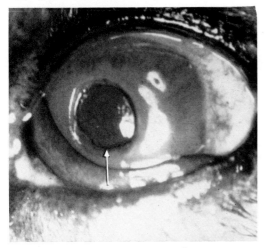

Fig. 90. Descemetocele.

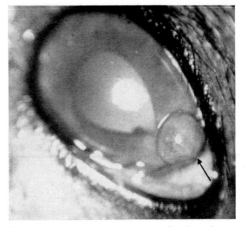

Fig. 91. Iris prolapse as a result of perforating injury to the cornea.

sary to effect a permanent bond (Par. 6:167).

6:115 An *iris prolapse* (Plate 6A and Fig. 91) is associated with loss of aqueous humor and temporary collapse of the anterior chamber. When a portion of the iris becomes entangled in the wound or protrudes beyond and adheres to the edges, the anterior chamber reforms. When the iris does not protrude beyond the normal curvature of the cornea, it becomes adherent either to the back of the cornea or fills in the space. When final healing is accomplished, an *adherent leukoma* results (Fig. 92A and B).

6:116 *Treatment.* If the iris protrudes beyond the cornea, this portion is disengaged from the wound and snipped off flush with the cornea (Fig. 93A, B and C). A protective conjunctival flap is then brought into place in the manner described (Par. 5:65) and aftercare is the same as that for des-

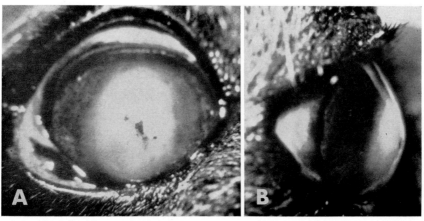

Fig. 92. Adherent leukoma. A. Front view. B. Side view.

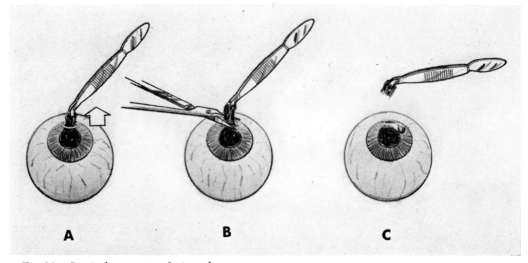

Fig. 93.   Surgical correction of iris prolapse.
A. Prolapsed portion disengaged from the opening. B. Prolapsed portion snipped off flush with the cornea. C. Appearance immediately following extirpation of the iris prolapse.

cemetocele (Par. 6:113). In the case of massive iris prolapse (Fig. 94), the eye should be enucleated.

6:117   A *staphyloma* is a bulging cicatrix lined by prolapsed iris. In other words, it is a protruding iris prolapse over which a fibrin film and layer of epithelium has formed. This in turn helps to create a seal between the iris and surrounding cornea. In this condition the cornea, in the prolapsed area, has been partially or nearly entirely destroyed.

6:118   *Treatment.* If the area is small

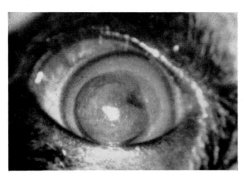

Fig. 94.   Massive iris prolapse.

and there remains a considerable portion of normal or near normal cornea, the prolapsed portion is handled in the manner described (Par. 6:116). If total (Fig. 94), the eye should be enucleated.

6:119   *Ectasia* (keratectasia) is a protrusion of the cornea alone resulting from chronic inflammatory changes with subsequent thinning of the structure. It may be due to softening of the cornea following interstitial keratitis. The bulging portion is opaque and conical in appearance (kerataconus). When fully developed, treatment is of no avail although a penetrating keratoplasty procedure could be considered (Par. 6:164).

Tumors of the Cornea

6:120   Neoplasms of the cornea rarely occur and almost always represent secondary extensions of lesions which are primary to some other part of the eye, *e.g.,* the uveal tract (Par. 7:62). Dermoid tumors have been discussed under congenital anomalies of the cornea (Par. 6:18).

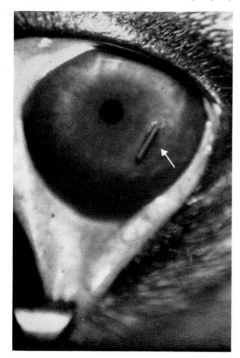

Fig. 95. Splinter embedded in cornea.

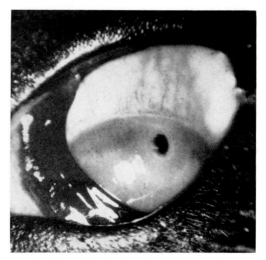

Fig. 96. Paint flake embedded in cornea.

Foreign Bodies of the Cornea

6:121 Foreign bodies, consisting of splinters (Fig. 95), thorns, awns, flakes of paint (Fig. 96) or metal, etc., may adhere or become embedded in the cornea causing pain, lacrimation and photophobia. A shot gun pellet may penetrate a cornea but usually becomes embedded in the posterior part of the globe or in the retrobulbar area. If the presence of a foreign body goes unnoticed or it is not removed, ulceration and/or edema and vascularization of the cornea may result. Excessive granulation tissue formation on the cornea may cover an embedded splinter (Plate 6B).

6:122 *Treatment.* When the foreign body is superficial, it can usually be removed under topical anesthesia in one of several ways. Useful instruments for this purpose include: an eyedropper to suck it from the surface; the point of a hypodermic needle or pointed blade to lift it from the cornea; or, eye splinter or dressing forceps to withdraw it.

6:123 When it is more firmly attached or has penetrated into the corneal stroma, it must be lifted or dug out with a spud (Fig. 97) or curette (Fig. 98). Deeply embedded splinters with a covering of epithelium must be "cut down on." Under general anesthesia and with the eye properly immobilized (Par. 6:135), an incision is made over the splinter with a No. 15 B.P. or No. 64 Beaver blade. It may then be removed by lifting. Care must be taken

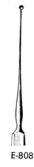

E-808

Fig. 97. Foreign body spud.

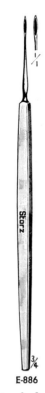

E-886

Fig. 98.   Foreign body curette.

not to perforate the cornea. Aftercare consists of a drop of atropine once a day and an antibiotic or sulfacetamide solution several times a day until re-epithelialization is well underway.

Wounds of the Cornea

6:124   Wounds may be non-penetrating or penetrating. Non-penetrating wounds and abrasions, though painful, heal readily (Par. 6:16) unless infected. Treatment consists of a drop of atropine once a day and an antibiotic or sulfacetamide solution several times a day until re-epithelialization is well under way.

6:125   Penetrating wounds of the cornea are subject to prolapse of the iris or injury to the deeper parts. If the perforating wound is limited to the cornea, the treatment then depends upon the extent of the laceration. Small

corneal perforations seal readily with quick reformation of the anterior chamber. The use of a conjunctival flap (Par. 5:65) and/or bandaging (Par. 3:81) following instillation of atropine and an antibiotic will immobilize the globe until a good seal is effected.

6:126   Extensive lacerations with collapse of the anterior chamber requires the careful placement of corneal sutures. If iris protrudes through the wound, it is safer to excise it (Par. 6:116) as no iris or foreign material should remain between the wound edges.

6:127   *Technique.* (*a*) The anterior chamber should be cleansed of any clots or debris. This may be accomplished by irrigating with sterile saline solution, using a lacrimal needle and syringe or irrigator. If the clot cannot be removed in this manner, sterile cotton wound toothpicks are used to roll the clot on (Par. 6:150). (*b*) Interrupted sutures of 6–0 silk, catgut, or mersilene attached to Greishaber needles (Par. 3:105) are placed so that they do not penetrate through the entire thickness of the cornea (Fig. 99A). This type placement prevents "wicking" from the anterior chamber. Eye tissue forceps or a special corneal forceps that prevents needle penetration (Fig. 100)* are used to grasp the corneal edges about 1 to 2 mm from the edge. The sutures must oppose the edges radially to avoid buckling. As many sutures are placed as are necessary to make the wound leak-proof. They are tied firmly but with care that sloughing of the corneal tissue will not occur. (*c*) An infusion of saline solution or an air bubble is made to reform the anterior chamber, prevent formation of anterior synechiae, and to check the snugness of the suture line

* Lawton Co., Inc., 435 4th Ave., New York, N. Y.

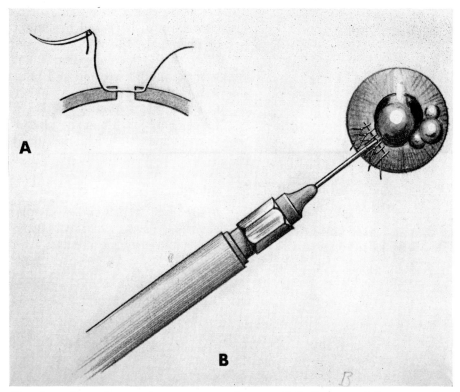

Fig. 99.   Corneal wound repair. *A.* Proper suture placement. *B.* Reformation of the anterior chamber by infusion of air bubbles. Lacrimal cannula and hypodermic syringe.

(Fig. 99B). (*d*) Following instillation of atropine and an antibiotic the lids may be sutured (Fig. 139, Chapter 9) and a bandage applied. If bandaging is not feasible, a supportive conjunctival flap (Par. 5:65) may be used.

6:128   Aftercare again should include atropine and a topical antibiotic. The corneal sutures are removed on the twelfth postoperative day.

Burns of the Cornea

6:129   Corneal burns produce pronounced subjective symptoms and, if neglected, may result in irreparable damage and loss of vision (Par. 3:22). Alkaline burns from detergents and soaps used in bathing are the most common types encountered (Plate 5F).

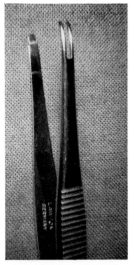

Fig. 100.   Special corneal forceps.

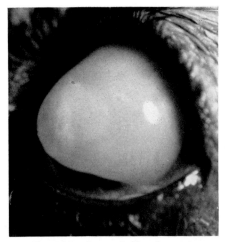

Fig. 101.   Severe bullous keratitis.

6:130   Regardless of whether the corneal burn is caused by lime, plaster, or chemicals, the eye and conjunctival folds should be immediately and copiously irrigated with normal saline solution or tap water as a first aid measure at home. Instillation of atropine for pain relief (Par. 3:27) and soothing preparations such as methylcellulose drops (Par. 3:90) usually suffice. An antibiotic to prevent secondary infection may be warranted.

6:131   Thermal and ultraviolet burns are treated symptomatically. Ether anesthesia burns (cone administration) are

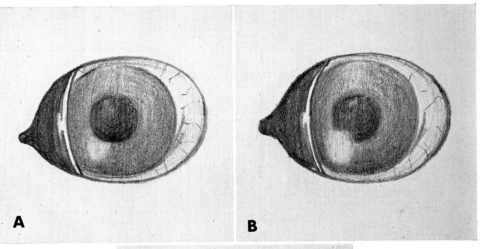

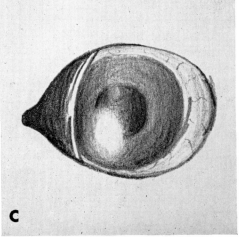

Fig. 102.   Corneal opacities according to density. *A.* Nebula. *B.* Macula. *C.* Leukoma.

best prevented by protecting the cornea with a bland ointment or castor oil (Par. 3:86).

Opacities of the Cornea

6:132   Lack of transparency of the cornea may result from inflammation, ulceration, or injury. A very small segment or the entire cornea may lose transparency. These opacities may be transient or permanent. Transient opacities are usually associated with healing in ulceration and injury and in superficial punctate keratitis (Par. 6:35). Permanent, dense opacities and scarring will be found in corneal dystrophies (Par. 6:38) and in the condition spoken of as adherent leukoma (Par. 6:115) (Fig. 92A and B). When the severe corneal edema associated with deep keratitis (Par. 6:76) subsides, the cornea will have a faint cloudiness throughout. The opacity and edema associated with bullous keratitis (Plate 5A) (Fig. 101) will clear with treatment, but a residual haze may remain.

6:133   According to density, a corneal opacity is called *nebula* (Fig. 102A) when faint and cloud-like; *macula* (Fig. 102B) when more pronounced and discernible as a gray spot in daylight; and *leukoma* (Fig. 102C) when dense and white.

6:134   *Treatment.* Topical steroids are helpful in hastening corneal clearing once an ulcer is healed. The opacity associated with corneal dystrophy is easily removed by performing a superficial keratectomy (Par. 6:152). Leukomatous scars are best left alone or, in the case of a show animal, tattooing (Par. 6:169) or a corneal transplant (Par. 6:164) can be considered. Opacity associated with deep keratitis can be minimized by using steroids by subconjunctival injection and topically. When the steroids fail to effect corneal clear-

ing, dionine (Par. 3:65) has, on occasion, proven useful.

Surgical Procedures of the Cornea

Fixation of the Globe

6:135   Often the clinician is prone to neglect performing a relatively simple procedure involving the cornea and associated perilimbal conjunctival structures because he has found it exceedingly difficult to fix the globe in a proper manner. The elasticity of the bulbar conjunctiva in all breeds, the natural recession of the globe in others, and the tendency for the eye to "roll back" under general anesthesia certainly contribute to this difficulty. Regardless of these facts, with proper instruments and a little practice, the eyeball can be fixed in any position to facilitate the performance of the desired procedure.

6:136   Instruments used are: a medium muscle (strabismus) hook, rat-toothed mosquito forceps, and eye fixation forceps (Fig. 103). With the use of

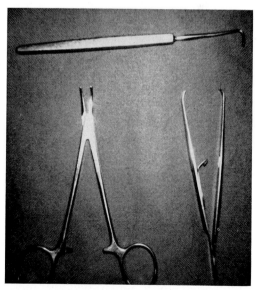

Fig. 103.   Instruments used for fixation of the globe; muscle hook, curved rat-toothed mosquito forceps, and fixation forceps (Graefe-spring catch).

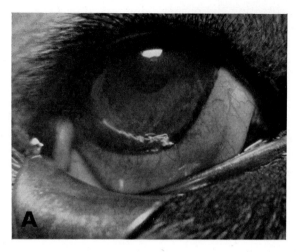

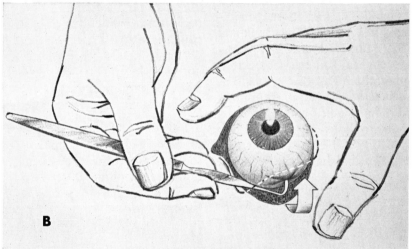

Fig. 104.   Preliminary step for proptosing of the globe. A. Muscle hook in position under the globe. B. "Cut-away" view.

the muscle hook it is possible to proptose a globe intentionally in order to start a superficial keratectomy properly. This smooths and renders taut the bulbar conjunctiva and minimizes hemorrhage in the vascular perilimbal area during the actual keratectomy procedure. The eyes of pekingese, pugs, Bostons, boxers, German shepherds, and cockers can be proptosed easily to facilitate the reaching of an area, and to smooth out the conjunctival folds when making incisions down to the sclera. In other breeds,

or when the palpebral fissure is small, a canthotomy (Par. 4:11) is first performed.

6:137   In the proptosing of a globe the muscle hook is inserted underneath the membrane nictitans, on the lower aspect of the globe, in the inferior rectus muscle area (Fig. 104A and B). Then, with pressure exerted in a lifting manner and spreading the lids with the other hand, the eye will proptose a reasonable distance beyond the lid margins. It can be fixed in this position by having an assistant continue to exert pressure with the hook and/or the rat-toothed mosquito forceps (Fig. 105A and B) or with the index finger (Fig. 106). Once the dissection of, for example, a pannus lesion or dermoid is well underway, the globe may be allowed to retract as the fixation forceps on the diseased tissue will suffice to control the eye for the continuation of the surgery.

6:138 There is no danger to the eye attending the proptosing procedure as the extraocular muscles allow for this "play" (Par. 1:20). However, proptosing of a globe should *never* precede or be used to fix the eye in an intraocular operative procedure.

6:139 The muscle hook is also used to rotate the eye in any desired direction. A slow, steady pressure is exerted to bring any aspect of the anterior portion of the eye into view. This facilitates peritomy (Par. 6:51), or the use of the beta-ray applicator at the limbus (Fig. 30, Chapter 3), and exposes the inferior aspect of the globe so that it might be grasped and held with rat-toothed mos-

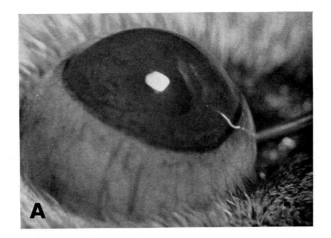

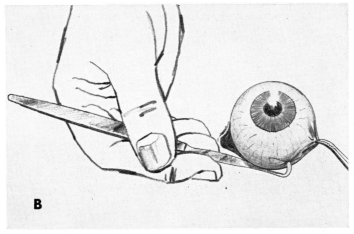

Fig. 105.   The proptosed eye. *A.* Muscle hook holding the globe. *B.* "Cut-away" view and additional fixation with rat-toothed mosquito forceps.

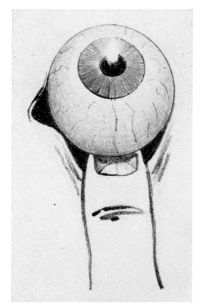

Fig 106.   Proptosed eye fixed with index finger.

quito forceps in preparation for, for example, paracentesis (Fig. 107).

6:140   Rat-toothed mosquito forceps will bite well into the bulbar conjunctiva and underlying episcleral tissue. This fixation alone or in conjunction with the eye fixation forceps placed on another part of the globe will be suffi-

cient to start the preparation of the conjunctival flap used in glaucoma and cataract surgery. Once a good flap is prepared, usually the fixation instruments can be released.

6:141   Stay sutures placed in either or both the body of the superior and inferior recti muscles can be used for globe fixation. This type of fixation is best suited to the human eye which has better extraocular muscle development. Vierheller[23] places a bridle suture in the tendon of the superior rectus muscle in intraocular procedures. The eye must be rolled downward. A small ½ circle needle is dipped through the conjunctiva about 12 mm back of the muscle tendon so that a loop of fine stitching material may be drawn around it. The ends of the bridle suture are then clipped to the drape under gentle traction.

6:142   Überreiter[24] uses stay sutures in this manner. The upper eyelid is pulled upwards by means of a lid retractor; the tendon of the superior rectus muscle is grasped through the conjunctiva with a muscle forceps and a stay suture is inserted beneath it with

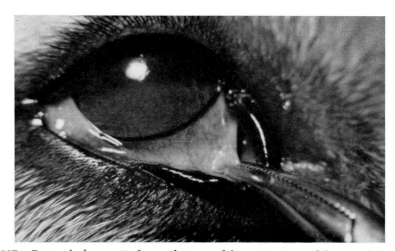

Fig. 107.   Rat-toothed mosquito forceps being used for positioning and fixation of the globe.

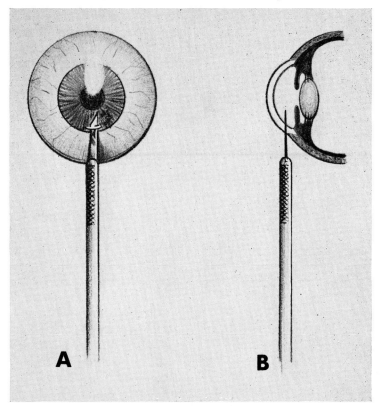

Fig. 108.   Paracentesis with pointed scalpel blade. *A.* Front view. *B.* Side view.

the aid of a full-curved needle. Similarly, a second stay suture is put into the interior surface of the membrane nictitans.

Paracentesis

6:143   Indications for paracentesis of the anterior chamber are: deep ulceration (Par. 6:107), ulcer with accompanying hypopyon (Par. 6:90), hypopyon alone (Par. 6:147), descemetocele (Par. 6:113), iritis (Par. 7:46), and hyphema (Par. 6:148). In addition to the mechanical release of the aqueous and any foreign substance contained therein, the fresh aqueous that subsequently forms to takes its place has a definite beneficial action on the disease process involved through increase in antibody titer[25] (Par. 7:9).

6:144   *Technique* (Fig. 108A and B). The puncture can be made with a special paracentesis needle (Fig. 109) or with a No. 11 B.P. blade or No. 65 Beaver blade. Short acting general anesthesia is required. After fixation of the eyeball (Fig. 107), the instrument is passed at a 45 degree angle to the surface through the cornea, 1 to 2 mm in-

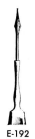

E-192

Fig. 109.   Paracentesis needle.

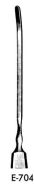

E-704

Fig. 110.   Iris spatula.

side the lower margin. The point of the blade should be parallel with the underlying iris. A sudden thrust type of puncture will insure a "clean" corneal incision and avoids the possibility of splitting corneal layers or pushing, rather than cutting through, Descemet's membrane. A 2 to 3 mm incision is sufficient for expelling aqueous alone. If further instrumentation is required to remove pus or blood clots, a larger incision and postplacing of one or more corneal sutures may be needed (Fig. 99A and B). When the knife tip has penetrated to the desired distance in the anterior chamber, the handle of the instrument is depressed, with pressure upon the posterior lip of the wound. It is then withdrawn slowly so as to evacuate the contents of the anterior chamber gradually. The beveled incision in the cornea will readily seal, and aqueous reformation of the anterior chamber takes place rapidly.

6:145   If it appears necessary to re-drain the anterior chamber the next day, an iris spatula (Fig. 110) may be used to reopen the wound. This can be safely done under topical anesthesia.

Hypopyon Drainage

6:146   Hypopyon is a collection of pus in the anterior chamber, consisting of polymorphonuclear leukocytes. The pus is an exudation from the iris and ciliary body when these parts participate in deep ulcerative keratitis or iritis. The pus collects at the bottom of the anterior chamber (Fig. 111) and may partially or completely fill this space. In the initial stages it may be of fluid consistency, but after existing for a time it is apt to have the addition of fibrin and forms a semi-solid, globular mass.

6:147   Upon performing a paracentesis, a fluid hypopyon will readily drain out or can be easily expelled by irrigation (Fig. 112). If in a semi-solid state, a dull iris hook and/or eye tissue forceps are used to bring the clot to the opening for withdrawal. The hook is inserted in the flattened position into the anterior chamber to the superior border of the mass (Fig. 113A). It is then turned to hook the border, and with a slow downward pull forces the lower part of the clot through the opening where it can be grasped and teased out with tissue forceps (Fig. 113B). At the least, this maneuver tends to break

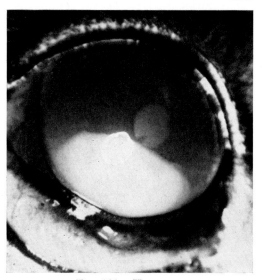

Fig. 111.   Hypopyon.

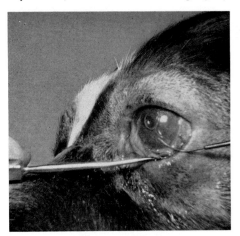

Fig. 112. Irrigation of the anterior chamber with sterile saline following paracentesis.

up the pus so that a part or all of it can then be expelled by irrigation. However, the presence of an organized hypopyon is not so important that a prolonged attempt to remove it might cause intraocular damage. The new aqueous

formation and the use of systemic enzymes (Par. 3:67) will hasten the absorption of what remains.

Hyphema Drainage

6:148   Hyphema is a collection of blood in the anterior chamber and occurs as the result of: injury to the globe; during the course of or following intraocular surgery; and in specific anomalies such as optic disc ectasia (Par. 11:72).

6:149   The blood may be in a constant fluid state as the result of capillary leakage, with continual drainage proceeding in a regular manner through the drainage plexus. In these instances a paracentesis will suffice to clear the anterior chamber but it quickly fills again with blood. The systemic administration of drugs which tend to decrease capillary permeability is necessary to help stop the leakage (Par. 3:88).

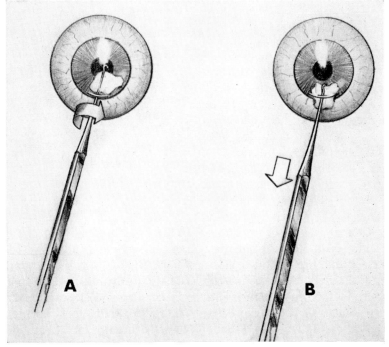

Fig. 113.   Removal of solid hypopyon from the anterior chamber. *A.* Iris hook engaging pus clot. *B.* Iris hook forcing pus clot to the opening.

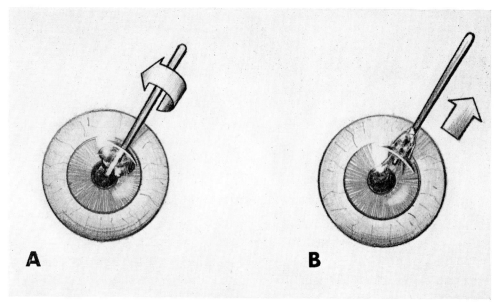

Fig. 114.   Removal of blood clots from the anterior chamber. *A.* Cotton wound toothpick engaging and rolling on clot. *B.* Withdrawal of the blood clot.

6:150   Hemorrhage into the anterior chamber following injury can be most serious. In the dog a clot forms quickly, it tends to organize and proliferate, often with a shrunken fibrotic globe resulting (phthisis bulbi). Immediately following injury with hyphema, atropine should be used in an attempt to prevent pupillary adhesions to the clot. If in twenty-four hours there has been no absorption and the clot occupies half or more of the anterior chamber, surgical removal is advocated. A paracentesis with sterile saline irrigation or the technique suggested for hypopyon drainage (Par. 6:147) may be found useful. Irrigation of the anterior chamber with a solution of fibrinolysin over a fifteen- to thirty-minute period is helpful in breaking up clots, but the present cost of this product often precludes its use. In most instances, it becomes necessary to enlarge the paracentesis incision sufficiently so that cotton wound toothpicks can be inserted into the chamber.

The clot will cling to and can be rolled onto the cotton and be removed in this manner (Par. 6:127) (Fig. 114A and B).

6:151   An even better technique for the removal of massive blood clots from the anterior chamber is to use the method described for entrance into the chamber under a conjunctival flap (Par. 9:139). In essence, a major intraocular procedure is often indicated if an eye is to be saved for both vision and cosmetic purposes.

Superficial Keratectomy

6:152   Removal of the superficial corneal layers is indicated for dermoids (Par. 6:19), advanced pannus (Par. 6:49), dystrophy (Par. 6:40), hyperplasia (Par. 5:57), stagnant or recurrent ulceration that does not involve Descemet's membrane (Par. 6:104), and scarring not associated with adherent leukoma.

6:153   The lamellar structure of the cornea (Par. 6:4) allows for a keratectomy at any level. I have adapted the following method as the safest, most practical way of removing the pathological tissue at a corneal level which will generally insure the finding of a perfectly clear stroma underneath.

6:154   *Technique* (Fig. 115A, B and C). Instruments required are: No. 64 Beaver blade or No. 15 B.P. blade; blunt tip, thin bladed tenotomy or strabismus scissors; eye tissue forceps; and, fixation forceps. The eye is first proptosed and immobilized to facilitate the procedure (Par. 6:137).

6:155   An incision is made through the conjunctiva and Tenon's capsule down to the sclera (Fig. 115A). The incision site is usually 1 to 2 mm from the limbus but is made at whatever distance from the limbus which may be required to include any accompanying conjunctival pathology. Having reached the scleral level, the operator now has a landmark and the proper level for the dissection.

6:156   The resection of the lesion is done in the manner of skinning an animal (Fig. 115B). The stroke of the blade is parallel with the line of cleavage and slight pressure is exerted with the flat of the knife against the scleral and, thence, the corneal surface. In the dissection to the limbus, the back edge of the point may be used. Upon reaching the limbus the sharp edge, held flat to the surface, must be used to shave through this very adherent structure (Par. 5:3). Upon reaching the cornea the rest of the peeling off advances quickly and easily. With a firm grip on the portion to be removed the proptosed eye may be allowed to return to the orbit. First, however, it is well to touch the bleeding points on the scleral side

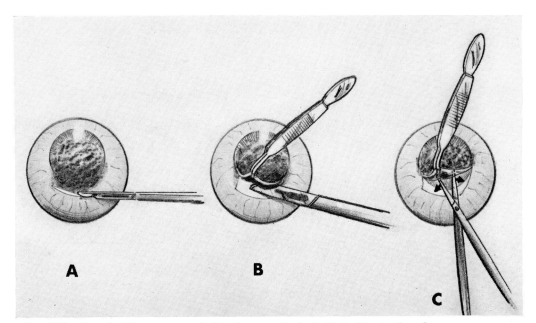

A   **B**   **C**

Fig. 115.   Superficial keratectomy. *A.* Initial perpendicular knife incision to the sclera.
B. Flat knife incision through the limbal area. *C.* Scissors used in spread fashion to separate lesion from clear cornea.

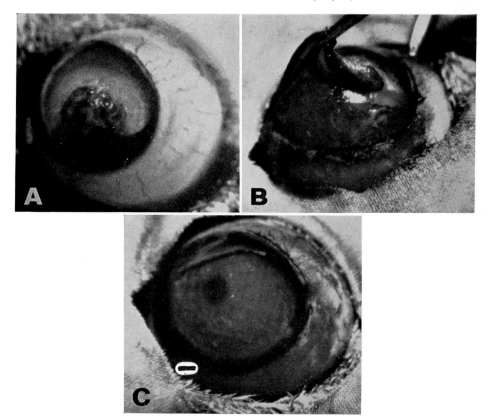

Fig. 116.   *A.* Eye afflicted with heavy pannus proptosed in preparation for superficial keratectomy.
B. Halfway through surgery. Note clear stroma under lesion being removed. *C.* Surgery completed. Note line of demarcation between normal intact cornea (upper one third) and area from which lesion was removed.

with either the electrocautery (Par. 3:73) or with a muscle hook that has been heated over an alcohol lamp.

6:157   The eye speculum is inserted for better exposure and the dissection is continued using either the back of the blade and/or the scissors in spread fashion (Fig. 115C). The scissors are also used to snip through this limbal margin, one blade on the corneal and the other on the scleral side. Irrigation with sterile saline is necessary to keep the structures moist and to wash away the blood and debris.

6:158   Finally, when the resection has reached normal tissue, the scissors

are used to cut the lesion from its base. Ordinarily, about one-half of the corneal thickness has been removed (Fig. 116A, B and C).

6:159   If one has made the original incision deep enough, the iris and pupillary margin are readily made out. Should this not be true and the corneal tissue is not clear, then either the incision has not reached the proper level or the scar or lesion involves the entire thickness of the cornea and cannot be successfully removed.[26] If the proper level has been reached (scleral landmark), it is seldom that a deeper opacity (Par. 6:40) will be encountered in the dog's cornea. In any event, a further level beyond this should not be sought since there is danger of puncturing the cornea.

6:160   If the lesion is limited to one segment of the cornea, it is not necessary to peel off the entire surface. Only the lesion and clear cornea a few millimeters beyond should be removed. The remaining healthy corneal tissue is instrumental in hastening regeneration of the area from which the lesion was excised (Par. 6:16). If the entire top layer needs to be removed, regeneration will nevertheless be complete. But it will take longer and will be accompanied by considerable vascularization and granulation.

6:161   Beta radiation at the completion of surgery is helpful in preventing too rapid an invasion of vessels and granulation tissue (Fig. 30, Chapter 3). Approximately 1500 r.e.p. administered at each area of the excised limbus will allow re-epithelialization to take place in a more orderly fashion.

6:162   *After care.* Following surgical procedure a drop of atropine and an antibiotic are instilled. The eye or eyes are bandaged (Figs. 117, 31) and a protective hood is placed (Fig. 45A). Ordinarily the bandage is removed the next day and the eye is treated "open" with atropine and the antibiotic. There is certainly no contraindication to daily bandage changes and the advantages have been elicited (Par. 3:80). However, if both eyes have been operated and are covered, there is the problem of ambulation. On the second or third day, when the cornea begins to epithelialize, it assumes a light milky hue and may give rise to fear that the operation has not been successful. At about the sixth postoperative day the cornea will appear somewhat more cloudy but is now re-

generated to the point that a topical steroid-antibiotic preparation can be started. The atropine is stopped. If excessive vascularization and granulation are noted, subconjunctival steroid injections (Par. 3:56) are indicated. A therapeutic vitamin capsule (Par. 3:64) is administered daily following surgery to enhance the corneal regeneration. The patient can usually be discharged on about the tenth postoperative day with the steroid-antibiotic preparation being used for only another week or so (pannus excepted) (Par. 6:47). The cornea will be healthy and clear in from two to four weeks following surgery.

6:163   I have not found it necessary to employ lamellar grafts to fill the corneal defect left by the excision. In fact, in several instances where a lamellar graft was used on one eye and the second left to regenerate naturally, the best end result was achieved in the second eye.

Corneal Grafts (Keratoplasty)

6:164   A few papers[22, 27–29] have been written on the use of partial (lamellar) and total (penetrating) corneal grafts

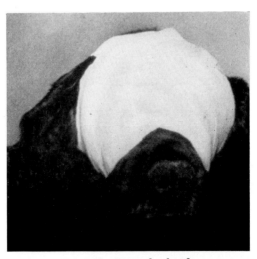

Fig. 117.   Binocular bandage.

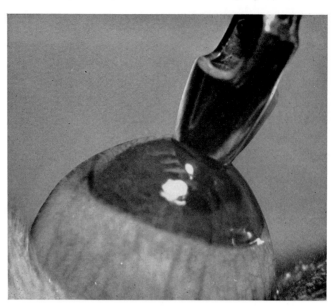

Fig. 118.   Trephining graft from donor eye.

in the dog. These investigators have concerned themselves primarily with the development of technique using normal corneas. Consequently, the indications for keratoplasty procedures for the dog have not been well established. It is apparent, however, that there would be few indications for the use of grafts in the dog as compared to man. Visual requirements differ, the dog's cornea is not subjected to extensive scarring, and one eye serves the dog well.

6:165   Of even more significance is the fact that the simple superficial keratectomy procedure (Par. 6:152) for the purpose of removing pannus lesions, dermoids, dystrophic areas, hyperplasia and superficial scars from the cornea is followed by natural corneal regeneration, thus negating the need for replacement grafts. As pointed out (Par. 6:163) the use of lamellar grafts may well complicate rather than help achieve satisfactory healing.

6:166   To establish indications for corneal transplantation in the dog, based

on results obtained, an accurate selection of cases is important since the graft may become involved in any concurrent pathology. For example, removal of a pigmented area from the cornea with the purpose of replacing that defect with a graft is destined to failure unless the cause of the pigmentation is eliminated and its re-entry to the graft prevented.

6:167   I am convinced that either lamellar or total grafts are helpful and that their use may be imperative in those instances in which a fistulous corneal lesion fails to fill in (Plate 5H). In cases of this type a descemetocele is present which will "seal over" for a period, only to rupture with leakage of aqueous. This process then repeats itself over and over. Both lamellar and full thickness grafts have been employed with uniformly good results. Direct suturing with 7–0 silk and 5 mm Greishaber needles is currently the method of choice. Four stay sutures are preplaced in the donor graft prior to its complete removal from the donor eye (Fig. 118). Eight or more additional sutures are required, depending upon the type of graft used. Additional support from a membrane nictitans flap and bandaging is necessary for the most uniform results. The corneal sutures should not be removed in less than fourteen days, although the flap can be released and daily bandage changes stopped at the end of the first week.

6:168   Keratoplasty procedures can be classified as highly specialized surgery. The indications are few, the instrument requirements and surgical astuteness are absolute. Enlisting the aid of a medical or veterinary ophthalmologist skilled in this field is obligatory.

Tattooing and Coloring

6:169   To remove the disfigurement in cases of dense scarring (adherent leukoma), tattooing of the area may be resorted to. Tattooing should not be considered before a firm scar has developed. Often by this time pigment migration (Par. 6:66) (Fig. 84) has served the purpose of obscuring the scar.

6:170   Special corneal tattooing needles and inks are available for this purpose. The ink paste is introduced into the cornea with a needle bundle using an oblique puncture technique. It is often necessary to repeat the procedure as the dye washes out in time.

THE SCLERA

Anatomy

6:171   The sclerotic coat (sclera) is the tunic which, with the cornea, forms the external fibrous layer of the eyeball and serves to maintain the form of the globe (Par. 1:14). The structure of the sclera is made up of a laminated pattern of fibrous tissue and elastic fibers. An outstanding feature of the dog's eye is the variation in thickness.[1] At the equator it is thin (0.28 mm), while in the ciliary region, it is much thicker (1.0 mm or more) and it has a well developed venous plexus. Around the optic nerve the sclera is again thicker (0.8 mm).

6:172   The sclera is punctured at several points for the passage of nerves and blood vessels. The head of the optic nerve is situated in the posterior wall and may be central, or it may be lateral or medial to the posterior pole. The part through which the nerve passes is known as the *lamina cribrosa*. Prince[1] points out that there is not an actual hole in the sclera, however. The scleral fibers separate and reduce in number until they form a fine screen through which the optic nerve fibers pass. This screen (lamina cribrosa) is the weakest part of the eye tunic. The limbal area of the sclera is pigmented laterally and medially, but not dorsally and ventrally.

6:173   Surrounding the sclera is the quite vascular episclera (Par. 1:16) which unites in the limbal area with the conjunctiva and sclera. Its main function is to provide nutrition to the outer parts of the almost avascular sclera.

Diseases

6:174   Affections of the sclera include inflammation, staphyloma, injuries, and extension of intraocular tumors. All occur infrequently.

6:175   *Episcleritis* (Plate 6D). A localized inflammatory lesion involving primarily the perilimbal area. The area is somewhat engorged, is nodular in appearance and feel, is immovable, and looks suspiciously neoplastic. The conjunctiva can be moved over it freely. Usually but one eye is involved. The course is chronic and there is a tendency for it to recur.

6:176   In man episcleritis is a disease of systemic origin. In the dog we have seldom been able to determine a specific cause, although a particular hypersensitivity is believed to play a role. Steroid therapy consisting of subconjunctival injections (Par. 3:56) at forty-eight-hour intervals and a follow-up with drops or ointment will allay the process and keep it under control. As mentioned, relapses are common and continual use of steroid preparations may be necessary. A transient periodic episcleritis lasting for a few hours to a few days has been observed in several instances.

6:177   *Staphyloma* or ectasia of the sclera occurs when the wall has been weakened by the buphthalmos of chronic glaucoma (Par. 9:31). In these instances the scleral wall becomes uniformly thin, takes on a "blue" appearance because of the underlying uveal tissue showing through, and may bulge in the weakened sections. Penetrating wounds and poor closure following a scleral incision into the anterior chamber in, for example, glaucoma and cataract surgery, also predispose to a localized staphyloma.

6:178   Treatment of scleral ectasia depends upon the cause. Glaucomatous eyes that have reached this stage are best enucleated. If the bulging is due to wounds or poor surgical closure, a repair may be made by incision, debridement (including excision of uveal tissue caught in the wound), tight suturing with catgut or 6–0 mersilene (Par. 3: 105), and accurate replacement of the episcleral tissues including Tenon's capsule and the conjunctiva. Scleral grafts and, recently, silicone implants have been used to replace and reinforce scleral tissue. The aftercare is similar to that described for wounds of the cornea (Par. 6:125).

6:179   *Injuries* usually occur as the result of bites and punctures from sharp objects or shotgun pellets. Penetrating wounds of the sclera, which result in

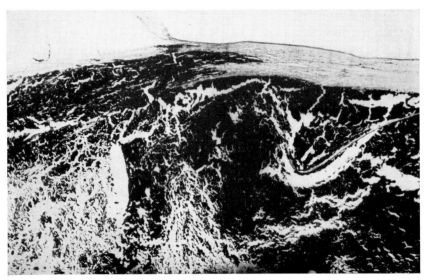

Fig. 119.   Scleral invasion of an intraocular melanoma.

loss of vitreous or are associated with an intraocular hemorrhage, usually end up in loss of the globe because of a subsequent panophthalmitis, or, the eyeball will become shrunken and fibrotic (phthisis bulbi) (Plate 8C).

6:180 An attempt should be made to preserve an eye by suturing the scleral and conjunctival wounds after excision of the prolapsed vitreous and uveal tissue. Small clean wounds often heal without reaction and merely require cleansing and the use of topical antibiotics. Radiographs of the head region are helpful in determining the presence and location of suspected pellets or foreign bodies, although they are usually allowed to remain if intraocular or in the orbit.

6:181 *Tumors* involving the uveal tract will, on occasion, extend into the sclera proper (Fig. 119). Enucleation of the globe and, possibly, the periorbital structures, should be performed to prevent systemic metastasis (Par. 7:77).

References

1. Prince, Jack H., Diesem, Charles D., Eglitis, Irma and Ruskell, Gordon L.: *Anatomy and Histology of the Eye and Orbit in Domestic Animals*, Springfield, Charles C Thomas, 1960.
2. Oda, Y. and Fukuda, S.: Electron Microscopic Studies on the Animals' Cornea, J. of Electronmicroscopy, *11*, 183–184, 1962.
3. Cello, Robert M.: The Pathology of Corneal Disease, A.A.H.A. Seminar, Los Angeles, 1962.
4. Magrane, William G.: Ocular Physiology—Clinical Application, No. Am. Vet., *36*, 388–389, 1955.
5. Magrane, William G.: Keratitis, Upjohn Veterinary Scope, *1*, #11, 1956.
6. Magrane, William G.: Vascularization—Its Significance in Diseases of the Cornea, J.A.V.M.A., *126*, 208, 1955.
7. Adler, Francis H.: *Physiology of the Eye*, 2nd ed., St. Louis, The C. V. Mosby Co., p. 41, 1953.
8. Allen, James H.: *May's Diseases of the Eye*, 23rd ed., Baltimore, The Williams & Wilkins Co., 1963.
9. Hogan, Michael J. and Zimmerman, Lorenz E.: *Ophthalmic Pathology*, 2nd ed., Philadelphia, W. B. Saunders Co., p. 311, 1962.
10. Überreiter, Von Otto: Ein besondere Keratitisform (Keratitis Superficialis Chronica) bein Hunde, Wien. Tierarztl. Mschr., *2*, 65–78, 1961.
11. Roberts, S. R.: The Nature of Corneal Pigmentation in the Dog, J.A.V.M.A., *124*, 208, 1954.
12. Michaelson, I. C.: Proliferation of Limbal Melanoblasts into the Cornea in Response to the Corneal Lesion, Brit. J. Ophth., *36*, 657, 1952.
13. Candlin, Frank T.: Catcott, Earl J. and Magrane, William G.: Beta-ray and X-ray Therapy in Diseases of the Eye, No. Am. Vet., *36*, 295, 1955.
14. Magrane, William G.: X-ray Therapy in Interstitial and Pigmentary Keratitis, No. Am. Vet., *29*, 582, 1948.
15. Catcott, Earl J. and Griesemer, R. A.: A Study of Corneal Healing in the Dog, Am. J. Vet. Res., *15*, 265, 1954.
16. Haggerty, T. E. and Zimmerman, L. E.: Mycotic Keratitis, So. Med. J., *2*, 153–159, 1958.
17. Ley, A. P.: Experimental Fungus Infections of the Cornea, Proc. Assoc. Res. Ophth., Am. J. Ophth., *42*, 49, 1956.
18. Smythe, R. H.: *Veterinary Ophthalmology*, London, Baillière Tindall & Cox, p. 248, 1956.
19. Smelser, G. K. and Ozanics, V.: Effect of Local Anesthetics on Cell Division and Migration, Arch. Ophth., *34*, 277, 1945.
20. Gundersen, M. T. and Liebman, S. D.: Effect of Local Anesthetics on Regeneration of Corneal Epithelium, Arch. Ophth., *31*, 29, 1944.
21. Wege, K.: Therapy of Virogenic Corneal Diseases with Gamma Globulin, Klin. Mbl. Augenheilk., *142*, 970–981, 1963.
22. Roberts, S. R.: A Feasible Technic for Corneal Grafting, Mod. Vet. Pract., *44*, 40–42, 1963.
23. Vierheller, Ralph C.: Cataract Surgery in the Dog, Mod. Vet. Pract., *43*, 45, 1962.
24. Überreiter, Von Otto: Examination of the Eye and Eye Operations in Animals, *Advances in Veterinary Science*, Vol. 5, New York, Academic Press, Inc., p. 52, 1959.
25. *Canine Surgery*, 4th ed., Santa Barbara, American Veterinary Publications, Inc., p. 332, 1957.
26. Weiner, Meyer and Scheie, Harold: *Surgery of the Eye*, 3rd ed., New York, Grune & Stratton, 1952.
27. Bernis, W. O.: Partial Penetrating Keratoplasty in Dogs, South-western Vet., *15*, 30–43, 1961.
28. Jensen, E. C.: Experimental Corneal Transplantation in the Dog, J.A.V.M.A., *142*, 11–21, 1963.
29. Lavignette, Andrew M.: Lamellar Keratoplasty in the Dog, Sm. An. Clinician, *2*, 183–197, 1962.

Chapter 7

DISEASES AND SURGERY OF THE IRIS AND UVEAL TRACT

Anatomy and Physiology

7:1   The second or vascular coat of the eye (uvea or uveal tract) lies beneath the sclera (Fig. 120). It consists of three parts which are intimately associated. In the anterior portion the *iris* is clearly visible and assumes a perpendicular position in the globe. The second component part (*ciliary body*) and the third (*choroid*) are both attached to the internal surface of the sclera. There is no distinct line of separation between the iris and ciliary body, but there is a marked junction of the ciliary body with the choroid. This area is known as the *ora ciliaris retinae* (*ora serrata in man*).

7:2   The *iris* (Fig. 121) consists of a spongy, connective tissue stroma, muscular fibers, and an abundance of vessels and nerves. It is covered anteriorly by endothelium and posteriorly by retinal pigment layers.

7:3   The two muscles present in the iris are the *sphincter* which encircles the pupil near its edge, and a *dilator* which extends from near the sphincter to near the iris root. The sphincter is the stronger of the two.

7:4   Purtsher[1] points out the significant differences between the iris of the dog and man. The canine iris possesses an immense arterial ring that is lacking in man. The peripheral part of the canine iris carries the important arteries and nerves that are intended for the ciliary body. Prince[2] states that the origin of this large vessel which forms a complete arcade around the iris is from the two long posterior ciliary arteries which reach it by passing right through the ciliary body. The dog appears to have a major, but no minor arterial arcade in the iris.

7:5   The iris regulates the amount of light admitted to the interior of the eye through the action of its pupil. The size of the pupil may vary among breeds and at different ages. Normally the pupil is in a state of constant change, with many factors operating which influence the size and movement. The behavior of the pupil during anesthesia has long been utilized to determine the depth of narcosis, a miotic pupil indicating stage 4 of surgical anesthesia. The tendency for the pupil to become small under anesthesia is so great that powerful mydriatics, when used preoperatively, often fail to prevent this miosis. The iris lies upon the anterior capsule of the lens when the pupil is contracted or moderately dilated. When fully dilated, it hangs free in the anterior chamber. The iris separates the *anterior* from the *posterior* chamber of the globe.

7:6   Most dogs' irides are brown or golden yellow with the pupillary border usually being more darkly pigmented. On its irregular posterior surface the iris is deeply pigmented with heavy radial striations. The color of the iris depends partly upon the variable pigment in the stroma cells and partly on that in the cells of the retinal layers. The depth of color of the iris plays a part in the reactions of the pupil to the various mydriatics. In the lightcoated breeds, with their corresponding lighter irides, the mydriatics are more prompt and long lasting in their effect.

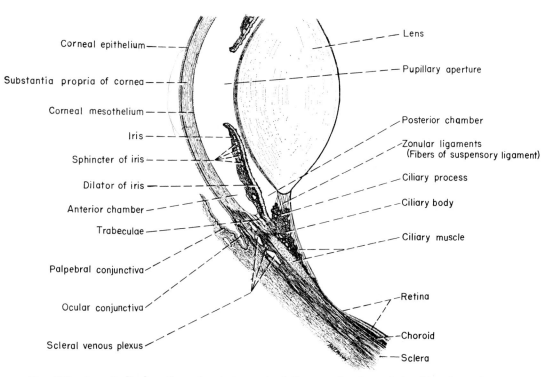

Fig. 120.   Longitudinal section of anterior part of the eye showing relationship of uveal tract to cornea and lens. (Miller, *Anatomy of the Dog*, courtesy of W. B. Saunders Company.)

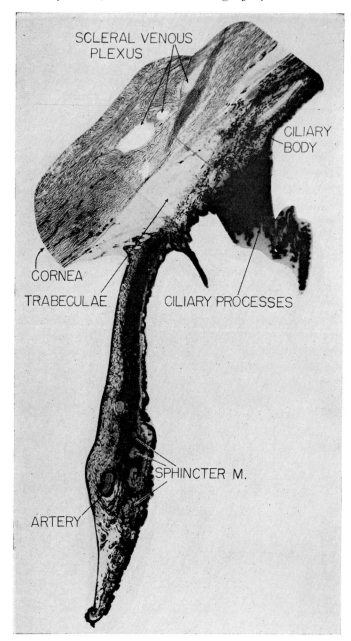

Fig. 121.   Iris and relationship to the drainage angle. (Prince *et al., Anatomy and Histology of the Eye and Orbit in Domestic Animals,* courtesy of Charles C Thomas.)

7:7   The *ciliary body* is that part of the vascular tunic which extends backwards from the base of the iris to the anterior part of the choroid. It consists of the ciliary *muscle* and the ciliary *processes.* The ciliary muscle is poorly developed as compared to man and this is probably the greatest factor in the limitation of the dog's accommodation (Par. 1:3). The ciliary body is richly supplied with nerves.

7:8   The ciliary processes range in number from 70 to 80. The larger processes extend to as much as 2.4 mm in length, while the smaller ones situated between them may show in a section as little more than half of this. Their width will usually be 0.14 mm.[2] It is on these ciliary processes that the fine suspensory or zonular ligaments (*zonules*), which hold the crystalline lens, have their attachments. The ciliary processes are important in that they secrete the nutrient fluid in the interior of the eye which, in turn, nourishes the cornea, lens and part of the vitreous. This fluid, the *aqueous* humor, under normal conditions, remains constant in amount and, by so doing, maintains a uniform intraocular pressure.

7:9   The aqueous is able to escape from the eye by way of the intrascleral plexus (Fig. 121), thus carrying the waste products of lens and corneal metabolism with it. If, for some reason, this escape channel is blocked, the intraocular pressure rises, with glaucoma as the result (Par. 9:41), since the aqueous continues to be secreted by the ciliary processes. The aqueous humor is a much more dilute fluid than blood serum and contains considerably less protein and a low concentration of specific immune bodies. If, however, the anterior chamber is subjected to draining by paracentesis, the fluid which refills the anterior chamber contains a high percentage of protein and shows a high titer of antibodies (Par. 6:143).

7:10   The *choroid* constitutes the third and final component of the uveal tract. It is placed between the sclera and the retina, extending from the ora ciliaris retinae to the opening for the optic nerve. The choroid is composed mainly of blood vessels and pigmented tissue and serves as a shield to absorb any light that passes through the retina or which is not reflected by the tapetum.

7:11   This vascular structure is bounded on either side by non-vascular membranes. Externally lies the suprachoroid, connected with the sclera by loose connective tissue. Underneath are several layers of large and medium sized anastomosing veins. Next comes a layer of capillaries (*choriocapillaris*) and, finally, *Bruch's* membrane lying between the choriocapillaris and the retina. The function then of the choroid is chiefly to serve as a nutrient organ for the retina, vitreous and lens.

7:12   The *tapetum* is a reflecting cellular layer of tissue situated behind the retina between the choriocapillaris and the larger vessel layer of the choroid. It serves to reflect light which has already passed through the retina, and to return it to the receptors so that they are doubly stimulated.[2] The tapetum (tapetum lucidum) varies in color and is responsible for the "eyeshine" so readily seen at night when the pupil is dilated and the dog stands facing a light.

The Pupil

7:13   The normal pupil is circular and regular and is larger in the dog than in man (Par. 1:5). The size should equal that of its fellow and both should respond alike to light stimulation (Par. 2:26). The movements of the pupil are contraction and dilatation.

7:14   The contracting fibers of the iris (sphincter) are supplied by the *third* nerve. The dilating fibers (dilator) are supplied by the *sympathetic*. Dilatation may be due to a decrease of third nerve tone or it may be due partially to stimulation of the dilator. Since the sphincter is the more powerful, the muscles are not equal antagonists. Contraction of the sphincter alone causes constriction of the pupil.

7:15   The rate of constriction varies (Par. 2:26), but the greatest part of the contraction occurs within the first few seconds and is completed within five or six seconds. When the light stimulus is removed, the pupil dilates quite slowly, the time for dilation being at least twice that required for contraction. Failure of dilated pupils to contract upon being subjected to light stimuli indicates a pathological condition (Par. 11:49), provided mydriatics have not been used prior to the examination.

7:16   Pupil contraction from light stimulation may be direct or consensual. A *direct* light reflex is obtained by exposing an eye to increased illumination and observing the resulting contraction. The *consensual* or indirect reflex is obtained by observing the contraction in the fellow eye when the first is subjected to light stimuli. These reactions should be practically equal. The consensual contraction is explained by the fact that the light stimulus in one eye is carried by the optic nerve and passes to both optic tracts and in this way to the nucleus of the third nerve of each side. Blindness in one eye abolishes the direct reflex in this eye, but its consensual reflex is preserved.[3]

7:17   A persistent dilatation is a significant symptom of glaucoma in the dog (Par. 9:24). This is usually unilateral, however, and is accompanied by the other diagnostic signs of increased intraocular tension. The dilatation of

progressive retinal atrophy is, in contrast, bilateral, and no other gross lesions are evident, ophthalmoscopy necessarily being employed as a diagnostic adjunct.

7:18   McGrath[4] points out that dilatation is seen also in paralysis of the oculomotor nerve, irritation of the cervical sympathetics, and as a common symptom of canine encephalitis. A miotic pupil may be seen in irritation of the oculomotor nerve, paralysis of the cervical sympathetics, and increased intracranial pressure (*e.g.*, brain tumors).

7:19   A pupil which may be of normal size and yet fails either to dilate or contract is highly suggestive of a posterior synechia (adhesion) of the iris to the anterior capsule of the lens (Par. 7:37). Iris atrophy, too, will result in an immobile pupil, the pupillary border of the iris, which possesses the sphincter fibers, being involved most conspicuously (Par. 9:36).

The Iris

7:20   *Congenital anomalies* of the iris include persistent pupillary membrane, heterochromia, polycoria, iris cysts, pigment spots or iris freckles and coloboma. These deviations from the normal are of interest but are only important from the standpoint of a differential diagnosis. No treatment is indicated or should be attempted.

7:21   *Persistent pupillary membrane* (Fig. 122). In the fetus the pupil is closed by a thin pupillary membrane. This membrane and its vessels are gradually absorbed before birth. When this absorption is incomplete, shreds or strands remain. These strands extend across the pupillary opening or, on occasion, can be found attached to an

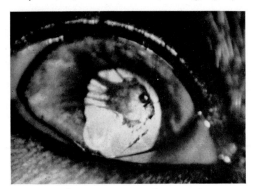

Fig. 122. Persistent pupillary membrane.

opaque spot on the anterior capsule of the lens (Par. 10:23).

7:22 *Heterochromia* (Plate 7A). Occasionally the two irides are of different color or part of one iris may differ in color from the rest of the iris. There does not appear to be any associated lack of visual acuity.

7:23 *Polycoria.* Rarely two or more pupils will be seen in one iris. To be a true polycoria each pupil must have its own sphincter fibers.

7:24 *Iris cysts* (Plate 7B). Pigmented cysts, resembling odd-sized cannon balls, may be found loose in the lower anterior chamber or adhered to the iris. If present in sufficient number, there may be some interference with vision. Iris cysts may also be acquired as a sequela to disease or degeneration of the iris. This acquired form should not be confused with the congenital type which is seen early and persists throughout the life of the dog.

7:25 *Pigment spots or iris freckles* (melanosis bulbi) appear as dark brown to black spots in and on the iris.

7:26 *Coloboma* of the iris is a notching which is usually present in the inferior half of the iris and is most often associated with coloboma of the cho-

roid. It can be considered very rare in the dog.

Iritis (Anterior uveitis) (Plate 7C)

7:27 Anterior uveitis refers to inflammations of the iris and ciliary body. Since inflammations of these structures are usually coexistent and cannot be differentiated on a clinical basis, those cases designated as iritis and cyclitis should be thought of as *iridocyclitis.* For the sake of convenience, I will use the term iritis when referring to an acute, recent involvement, and uveitis to indicate the chronic form of the disease.

7:28 *Etiology.* Iritis usually follows or accompanies some systemic disorder. It is most important that considerable time be expended in careful history taking and in conducting a thorough physical examination, including laboratory tests, if a cause is to be determined. Even then, the cause of the majority of those cases presented will never be known. The source often depends upon a toxin derived from a septic focus in some part of the body. This includes, for example, infected tonsils, teeth, prostate, sinuses, and pyometra. A classical chronic form of the disease has been seen as the result of toxoplasmosis and blastomycosis without obvious systemic symptoms. But, as Krawitz[5] indicates, although systemic disease may trigger a uveitis, the greater number of cases cannot be correlated to such disease. The present concept places the involvement of the anterior uvea as an allergic reaction excited by pathogens elsewhere. The resultant tissue reaction within the uveal tract most likely follows the classical concept of the antigen-antibody reaction mechanism. The exact cause, or initiating antigen, is usually obscure; therefore, the incrimination of a single specific agent is difficult.

7:29 Specific diseases such as distemper, leptospirosis, and hepatitis may, in turn, initiate an iritis. The "blue eye" (corneal opacity) following a hepatitis attack stems from an iridocyclitis which, in turn, is caused by the hepatitis virus. Carmichael's[6] study showed that during the acute febrile stage of hepatitis there was a mild anterior uveitis without corneal involvement. The corneal opacity supervened during convalescence. Two fundamentally different modes of pathogensis are postulated for the ocular lesions of the disease. During the acute phase of illness, prior to the onset of circulating antibodies, uveitis occurs that is related directly to effects of viral growth in vascular endothelium, and in reticuloendothelial elements of the anterior uvea. The severe iridocyclitis with corneal opacification that occurs in clinically recovered dogs possesses characteristics of the Arthus-type of ocular hypersensitivity.

7:30 A *traumatic* iritis occurs as a result of accidental injury or following intraocular surgery. The seriousness and course depends upon whether infection takes place.

7:31 A *secondary* iritis, following inflammation of adjacent tissues, may be found in severe corneal ulceration (Par. 6:90), lymphosarcoma (Par. 12:37), (Plate 6H), and in neoplasia involving the uveal tract.

7:32 *Subjective symptoms.* The ciliary blood vessels are congested and can be differentiated from injected conjunctival vessels (Par. 5:16). The cornea may have an overall haze. This is due to the possible presence of keratitic precipitates (leukocytes) clinging to the endothelium and, also, to the fact that

damage to the endothelium has allowed aqueous infiltration with its resultant corneal edema (Par. 6:12). The contents of the anterior chamber show changes. There is frequently turbidity (*aqueous flare*) which, when viewed obliquely, can be likened to the dust particles seen in a room when the drapes are pulled and a ray of sunshine pours in. In some instances great numbers of leukocytes and exudate from the iris may pour into the anterior chamber producing hypopyon (Fig. 111), (Chapter 6).

7:34 The iris itself looks spongy, muddy, and lusterless. Its color may alter some as the result of the congestion and exudation of cells and fibrin into its substance. The pupil is contracted (*miosis*) as a result of the distention of the radial blood vessels and irritation of the sphincter muscle. If the pupil is both miotic and irregular, adhesions between the posterior surface of the iris and the anterior capsule of the lens (*posterior synechia*) should be suspected. Although the tension of the globe in iritis is usually normal or below (*hypotony*), the presence of a posterior synechia can result in a secondary glaucoma (Par. 9:70).

7:35 *Course.* When an attack of iritis is acute and is diagnosed and treated early, the response is most dramatic and a "quiet" eye can be expected within several days to a week. If, on the other hand, the history and objective symptoms indicate a chronic condition, response to the best therapy is slow, and serious complications (Par. 7:36) can develop at any time, necessitating a change of medication or surgical intervention. Certain forms of iritis have a tendency to recur. Relapses are common because of the irritation effects of sequelae but probably more to the fact that the etiological factor has not been eliminated.

7:36   *Sequelae.* The usual complications following an attack of uveitis include: posterior synechiae, a cloudy film deposit upon the anterior lens capsule, complete seclusion of the pupil, occlusion of the pupil, iris atrophy, secondary glaucoma, vitreous opacities, lens opacities (cataract), and chorioretinitis. An endophthalmitis (Par. 7:53) may develop with loss of the eye.

7:37   A partial posterior synechia is of little consequence to the dog, but if a complete synechia with seclusion of the pupil occurs (*iris bombé*), (Plate 7D), a secondary glaucoma may result. When the iris is bound down throughout its entire pupillary margin (Fig. 123), there is a loss of communication between the anterior and posterior chambers. Thus the aqueous secreted by the ciliary processes (Par. 7:8) is retained in the posterior chamber rather than being able to escape through the pupillary opening, thence to the anterior chamber, and into the filtration angle and drainage system for the eye. The force of the aqueous in the posterior chamber causes the iris to billow forward creating the iris bombé.

7:38   Occlusion of the pupil is a filling in of the pupillary space with an opaque exudate or the entire iris may appear to obliterate the pupil area. Atrophy of the pupillary border and other sections of the iris stroma (Plate 7E) can, in turn, produce a secondary glaucoma because the sloughing pigment and iris debris clogs the drainage system.

7:39   Vitreous strands and debris may persist for some time or forever, and latent lens opacities can be expected in the chronic, recurrent forms

of uveitis. Chorioretinitis as a sequela is discussed in paragraph 11:25.

7:40   *Treatment.* Because of the serious complications and sequelae associated with this disease, appropriate therapeutic measures cannot be overemphasized.

7:41   The first consideration should be to alleviate the pain and get the inflammatory process under control. Determination of and elimination of the etiological factor, whenever possible, is of importance, but no time must be lost in "putting out the fire," with the cause as the secondary consideration.

7:42   Atropine (2 to 4 per cent) diminishes congestion of the iris, exerting a sedative action by paralyzing the ciliary body, and prevents adhesions by its mydriatic action (Par. 3:26). In the

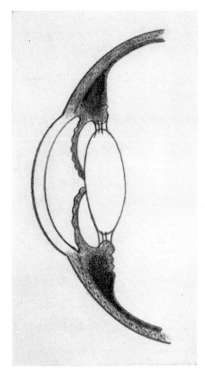

Fig. 123.   Anterior section of the eyeball showing posterior synechia (iris bombé).

initial stages atropine should be used every few hours, or until the pupil dilates well, and then twice a day. When the inflammation is severe, the pupil will not dilate readily and it may be necessary to make a subconjunctival injection of a drop or two of atropine combined with an equal amount of 10 per cent phenylephrine HCL (Par. 3:30). If the pupil fails to budge, a synechia is probably present.

7:43   Steroids, like atropine, are specific for treatment. A subconjunctival injection (Par. 3:56, Fig. 27) of a prednisolone preparation, repeated at forty-eight-hour intervals, will afford the best control of the inflammation. Topical preparations in the usual combined form may be helpful, and a single systemic administration (prednisone intramuscularly) is certainly not contraindicated.

7:44   Foreign protein injections have long been used in uveitis with variable results. With the advent of the steroids, their use has diminished but in specific stubborn cases they may still be found useful (Par. 3:69).

7:45   Systemic antibiotics and chemotherapy should be instituted in every severe case and where examination has disclosed a systemic foci of infection. It is extremely important, however, that the clinician is aware of the penetrating properties into the eye and through the blood aqueous barrier of the various antibiotics (Par. 3:40), else there will be no effect from their administration. Chloramphenicol (Par. 3:44) and the more lipoid-soluble sulfonamides are known to reach the aqueous of the eye in amounts sufficient to be of value.

7:46   Paracentesis of the anterior chamber (Par. 6:143) may be performed in every case of iritis to shorten the course of the disease, but its use becomes almost imperative in a uveitis that is not responding. A new plasmoid aqueous soon replaces the stagnant, and with its increase in antibody titer (Par. 7:9) will often reverse the course of the disease. If a hypopyon is present, a paracentesis will serve to expel this exudate from the anterior chamber (Par. 6:146).

7:47   Some relief from the pain and photophobia can be attained by keeping the patient out of bright areas and by the administration of salycilates. Moist, hot compresses diminish the pain and inflammation (Par. 3:71). Hospitalization is to be recommended, at least for that period necessary to complete the physical examination and bring the acute stage under control.

7:48   *Treatment of sequelae.* To repeat an old cliché, the best treatment is prevention. If, however, a posterior synechia results in a secondary glaucoma, an iridectomy (Par. 7:81) will

Plate 7.

A. Heterochromia.

B. Iris cysts.

C. Acute iritis. Note exudate in anterior chamber opposite 1:00 o'clock; dull, lustreless iris; and miotic pupil.

D. Iris-bombé and atrophy of the pupillary border. Note gray plastic exudate on the anterior capsule of the lens.

E. Iris atrophy and secondary glaucoma.

F. Cavernous hemangioma of the iris (entire upper half).

G. Malignant melanoma of the iris and ciliary body. Extension from 11:00 to 2:00 o'clock.

H. Malignant melanoma of the uveal tract with secondary glaucoma.

Plate 7

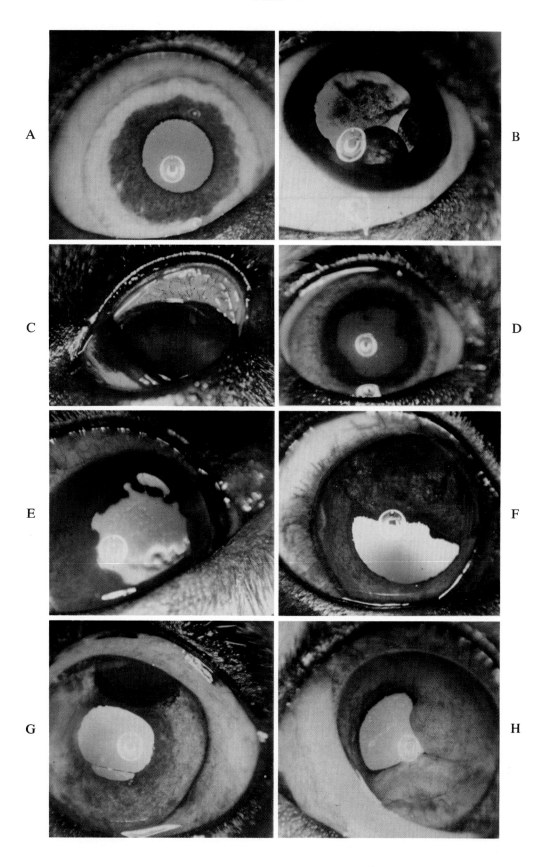

ordinarily re-establish communication between the posterior and anterior chambers. Iris atrophy and secondary glaucoma will probably necessitate the performance of a filtering procedure (Par. 9:107). Vitreous opacities may be minimized by instituting enzyme therapy (Par. 3:67). Lens opacities may be disregarded if vision is satisfactory in either of the two eyes. The damage resulting from chorioretinitis is permanent. Enucleation may be necessary in an endophthalmitis, but massive doses of, for example, chloramphenicol should be tried first (Par. 7:56).

Choroid

7:49   The only significant congenital anomaly of the choroid is the absence of the tapetum, thus exposing the choroidal circulation to ophthalmoscopic view (Par. 2:60, Plate 11H). In man, a similar condition (albinism), describes a congenital and hereditary deficiency of pigment and is associated with lowered visual acuity. If there is a loss of visual acuity in the dog with this anomaly, it has not been readily apparent.

Choroiditis

7:50   When posterior uveitis occurs in conjunction with or as an aftermath to an envolvement of the iris and ciliary body, it is not recognizable without the use of the ophthalmoscope. If the ocular media is not clear, and it usually is not in uveitis, then it remains for clearing to occur before ophthalmoscopy can be employed to assess the choroidal damage.

7:51   *Etiology.* Any cause listed for anterior uveitis (Par. 7:28) must be considered. Many obscure cases may be caused by *Toxoplasma.* Heeley's[7] work is conclusive as regards the important

role this organism plays in the cause of diffuse choroiditis and chorioretinitis.

7:52   *Treatment* of choroiditis in the active stage will be as recommended for uveitis in general (Par. 7:40). If a specific etiological agent such as Toxoplasma is responsible, sulphamethazine and Daraprim therapy has proven useful. As mentioned before, the damage resulting from chorioretinitis is permanent.

Endophthalmitis

7:53   This disease is also known as purulent uveitis and is an infection of the interior of the eye by pyogenic organisms. The infection may be of either internal or external origin.

7:54   *Symptoms.* In the initial stages the purulent exudate fills the vitreous, often with little or no external evidences of inflammation. A dirty yellowish reflex is obtained from the interior of the eye. Within a short time the purulent exudate fills the whole interior, with pus in the anterior chamber, and all the symptoms of an acute uveitis most apparent. The patient exhibits considerable pain, is generally ill, and shows conjunctival congestion, chemosis, lid swelling, and a cloudy, vascularized cornea. When all structures of the eye are involved, the condition is referred to as a *panophthalmitis.*

7:55   If treatment fails or an enucleation is not performed, the purulent mass degenerates, the eyeball softens and the process ends with atrophy of the eyeball (*phthisis bulbi*) (Plate 8C).

7:56   *Treatment.* Regardless of the stage or severity it is usually impossible to save any vision. If diagnosed early, and before the whole eye is involved, an occasional eye might be preserved for cosmetic purposes following para-centesis, intravitreal and subconjunctival antibiotic injections, and maintenance of a high therapeutic level of the systemic sulfonamides and chloramphenicol. When iris-lens adhesions are present, and this is generally the case, an iridectomy (Par. 7:81) will serve to re-establish intraocular circulation and will afford a pathway for the antibiotic instillation and irrigation of the posterior and vitreal chambers. Penicillin G (crystalline-potassium) (1,000,000 units) in 5 cc of sterile saline solution has been used successfully for this purpose.

7:57   If the combination of surgery and systemic antibiotic therapy fails to alleviate the symptoms described, with noticeable improvement within several days, an enucleation should be performed.

Sympathetic Ophthalmia

7:58   Involvement of a normal eye with a serous or plastic inflammation of the uveal tract due to the effects of a similar inflammation in the first eye is referred to as sympathetic ophthalmia. It is not known to occur in the dog, as it does in man, nor has there been given a satisfactory explanation for this difference.

7:59   Sympathetic ophthalmia, as it occurs in man, should not be confused with sympathetic irritation in which the unaffected eye of the dog waters more than usual and may exhibit some photophobia.

Injuries

7:60   Injuries to the iris and uveal tract may be of the perforating or non-perforating type. In perforating wounds of the globe, in which there is an iris prolapse, the prolapse should be excised

(Par. 6:116). Lacerations of the sclera, with prolapse of a part of the uveal tract, may need to be sutured following excision (Par. 6:127).

7:61   Non-perforating injuries (concussion) may cause a transient or permanent mydriasis from paresis or paralysis of the motor nerve fibers supplying the sphincter and the ciliary muscle. Concussion can cause an *iridodialysis*, a separation of the iris from the ciliary body. In these instances a black cresentic area will be noted at the site of detachment and there will be some displacement of the corresponding pupillary border. This type of injury usually produces an accompanying hyphema (Par. 6:148).

Tumors

7:62   Tumors of the iris and uveal tract include benign melanoma, cysts, hemangiomas, epitheliomas, and malignant melanomas.

7:63   Although of uncommon occurrence, uveal tumors in the dog cannot be considered rare even though comparatively few intraocular tumors have been documented in the veterinary literature of the world. The following text is in summary of my series.[8]

Literature

7:64   Saunders and Barron (1958), in a survey of the world literature, found less than 50 reports of intraocular tumors of any kind and these included all animals. They have reviewed 15 cases of primary pigmented intraocular tumors in the dog. Eleven of these were from the files of the Armed Forces Institute of Pathology, and three from individual contributors. Two additional primary nonpigmented intraocular tumors in the dog and one in the cat are the subject of a second paper (Barron and Saunders 1959). Aside from these works, there appears to be no general discussion of intraocular tumors of animals in the literature. Most of the authors cited by Saunders and Barron believed that the tumors they were reporting were very rare. Smythe (1956) briefly mentions seeing melanotic sarcomas of the uveal tract in a few reddish-colored dogs such as airdales. Grice and Hutchison (1960) described a retinoblastoma, a congenital malignant tumor arising from the nuclear layers of the retina. On clinical examination it was thought to be a malignant melanoma. Überreiter (1959) records a sarcoma of the iris.

7:65 Malignant melanoma of the uveal tract is by far the most common malignant intraocular tumor found in man, and occur mostly in advanced middle age (Hogan and Zimmerman 1962) (Reece 1956). Those involving the iris alone comprise approximately 5 to 8 per cent of all uveal melanomas. Iris melanomas rarely metastasize and mortality is much less than in similar tumors of the ciliary body or choroid. Being easily seen they are ordinarily removed at an early stage.

7:66 In a necropsy study of over 2000 eyes (man) with malignant melanomas of the uveal tract, it was found that in 21 per cent of the affected eyes the media were opaque at the time of enucleation. Thus the tumor could not be visualized clinically. In 11 per cent of these eyes proved to contain malignant melanomas of the choroid or ciliary body, there was not even the clinical suspicion of the presence of an intraocular neoplasm. In more than 90 per cent of such unsuspected melanomas, the eye was glaucomatous (Makley and Teed 1958).

Cases

7:67 Within a nine-year period, I saw two cases of benign primary non-pigmented and seven cases of malignant primary pigmented intraocular tumors. Of these nine, three were described in the Saunders-Barron papers.

7:68 These cases were received mostly by referral and are certainly not to be considered common in occurrence. However, it became evident in the study that neither should they be considered rare because; 1. in most instances either no diagnosis or an erroneous diagnosis had been made, 2. similar cases are known to have been euthanized because of blindness or discomfort without a diagnosis being established, and 3. of the incidence of intraocular new growths reported in man. Nine different breeds were represented in the total series (9) and the age ranged from eight to twelve years.

1. *Benign non-pigmented*

7:69 Two cases of non-pigmented tumors were; 1. a cavernous hemangioma of the iris and 2. an epithelioma of the ciliary processes.

7:70 The hemangioma involved the entire upper half of the iris and filled the upper anterior chamber (Magrane 1954) (Plate 7F). Progressive in nature, vision was about to be lost because of filling of the pupillary space.

7:71 The epithelioma (round 6 mm nodule) was visible on pupil dilatation. It occupied the posterior chamber on the temporal side, was crowding against the lens, and pushing the iris forward.

7:72 In both instances a uveal melanoma was suspected, but exploratory surgical intervention proved to be completely successful. In rather delicate lengthy procedures, each of the two eyes was saved with normal vision resulting.

7:73   Hemangiomas of the iris must be considered rare in occurrence since only a few have been reported in man. Epitheliomas, which arise from the non-pigmented epithelium of the ciliary processes, are more common, but are usually found accidentally in the microscopic examination of eyes removed for other causes in the human. To my knowledge neither of these two tumors have been otherwise reported in the dog.

7:74   The important aspect of these two cases is the similarity of the gross clinical findings with malignant melanoma of the uveal tract. Yet the prognosis for preservation of vision and the globe itself is at near opposite extremes.

2. *Malignant pigmented*

7:75   Of the seven primary pigmented tumors, six were confirmed malignant melanomas. In the seventh, an involvement of apparently only the ciliary body, a definite diagnosis was not established, but it was thought to be either a diktyoma or medullo-epithelioma (carcinoma).

7:76   In each instance only one eye was involved and the growth observable in the iris was usually an extension from the remainder of the uveal tract (Plate 7G). A secondary glaucoma resulting from drainage angle occlusion by the tumor was either present at the time of the initial examination or followed with continued progression of the growth. It became necessary eventually to enucleate six of the seven eyes with malignant tumors. In the seventh, it appeared on gross clinical examination that only the iris was involved. An iri-

dectomy, including the lesion, was performed with no extension or recurrence discernible eighteen months following surgery.

7:77   A complete follow-up until death was not possible in each instance, but the malignant nature of the primary intraocular growth was demonstrated in the case of a male, eight-year-old cocker spaniel. Two-thirds of the iris was involved and the growth extended anteriorly to the cornea (Plate 7H). A secondary glaucoma was present. The fundus was normal. The eye was enucleated and histologically the growth was found to involve the iris and ciliary body and was classified as a highly malignant melanoma of the epitheloid type. Eight months later euthanasia was performed because of a progressive respiratory involvement and rapid tumorous enlargement of the upper gum. Generalized metastasis to the nasal sinuses, turbinates, lungs, stomach and adrenal gland were noted.

7:78   In each of the eyes examined the cornea was clear and recognition of the new growth was not difficult. Aids to recognition included one or more of the following:
1. an irregular pupil or loss of pupillary space;
2. filling in of a part of the anterior chamber and drainage angle;
3. increased pigmentation of the part;
4. iris thickened and/or thrown into irregular undulating folds;
5. episcleral congestion and increase in tension;
6. scleral ectasia opposite the ciliary lesion.

7:79   Each case of intraocular new growth must be evaluated on an individual basis. In the very old it may be best to postpone enucleation until such time that a secondary glaucoma and discomfort to the animal makes it necessary. Melanomas of the uveal tract are known to metastasize slowly in most instances. Thus, early enucleation would only be imperative in the young to middle aged dogs. If only the iris appears to be involved, an iridectomy may well save vision and a globe. If, on the other hand, at the time of surgical procedure or sometime following, it is learned that there is further invasion of the uveal tract, there still remains the alternative of enucleation.

Surgery of the Iris

7:80   Surgical excision of iris prolapse is the most commonly performed procedure. This has been described (Par. 6:116).

7:81   *Iridectomy,* excision of a portion of the iris is often performed in both cataract and glaucoma surgery. Because of the nature of the iris in the dog, a profuse hemorrhage usually follows the cutting or removal of a portion of the iris (Par. 7:4). For this reason

I routinely use the electrocautery (Par. 3:73) to perform an iridectomy.

7:82   An iridectomy will be complete or peripheral depending upon the type condition being operated on. For example, a complete iridectomy, which includes removal of a segment from the pupillary border to the base of the iris, would be the surgical procedure of choice in an iris-lens adhesion (iris bombé) (Plate 9H). A peripheral iridectomy (Plate 9G) may be performed in an acute congestive glaucoma (Par. 9:104). This type of iridectomy is more appropriately referred to as a basal iridectomy since it involves the iris base. A pupillary iridectomy is routinely used to afford more working space in cataract extractions (Par. 10:88).

7:83   In nearly every instance a limbal based conjunctival flap is prepared prior to the section into the anterior chamber and performance of a complete iridectomy. One or more preplaced sutures (Par. 9:137) are usually used. Following the section into the anterior chamber, the iris is withdrawn

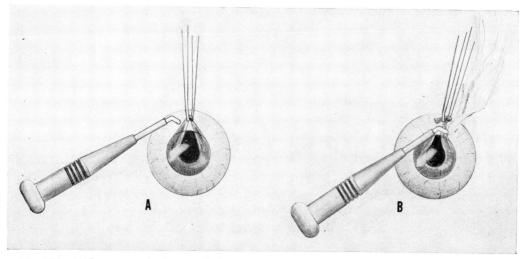

Fig. 124.   Iridectomy with electroscalpel. A. First cut from base to pupillary border. B. Completing excision of iris wedge.

with a dull iris hook, eye tissue forceps, or iris forceps. With the assistant holding the conjunctival flap out of the way, the electroscalpel is used to complete the iridectomy (Fig. 124).

7:84   If a peripheral iridectomy is to be performed, a small curved iris forceps is barely introduced into the anterior chamber, the surface of the iris is grasped just beyond its base and pulled just far enough into the wound so that the bottom of the forceps escapes the wound margin. The electroscalpel can then be used to excise a portion of the base, although extra caution must be exercised to avoid burning the surrounding structures. If either the electroscalpel or small curved iris scissors are used for the cutting, the excision should be as close as possible to the iris forceps so as to include in the cut only that part of the iris close to its base, thus avoiding the cutting of the iris sphincter.

7:85   As with any and all specialized intraocular procedures mentioned in this book, the reader is urged to pursue the technique further in one or more of the splendid, well-illustrated ophthalmic surgery texts and to enlist the aid of an ophthalmic surgeon in his initial attempts.

References

1. Purtscher, C.: The Large Arteries of the Canine Iris, Berl. U. Munch. Tierärzt. W. Schr., *74*, (22), 436–438, 1961.
2. Prince, Jack H., Diesem, Charles D., Eglitis, Irma and Ruskell, Gordon L.: *Anatomy and Histology of the Eye and Orbit in Domestic Animals*, Springfield, Charles C Thomas, 1960.
3. Allen, James H.: *May's Diseases of the Eye*, 23rd ed., Baltimore, The Williams & Wilkins Co., 1963.
4. McGrath, John T.: The Neurologic Examination of the Dog with Some Clinico-Pathologic Observations, University of Pennsylvania Vet. Ext. Quart., *54*, 5–47, 1953.
5. Krawitz, Leonard: Disease of the Anterior Uvea of the Dog, J.A.V.M.A., *144*, 988, 1964.
6. Carmichael, L. E.: The Pathogenesis of Ocular Lesions of Infectious Canine Hepatitis, Path. Vet., *1*, 73–95, 1964.
7. Heeley, D. M.: Toxoplasmosis, J. Sm. An. Prac., *4*, 435–446, 1963.
8. Magrane, William G.: Tumors of the Eye and Orbit in the Dog, Proceedings XVIIth World Veterinary Congress, Hanover, Germany, *2*, 1095–1098, 1963.

Chapter 8

DISEASES AND SURGERY
OF THE ORBIT

Anatomy

8:1   Prince[1] describes the canine orbit in somewhat the following manner. The shape of the head has some influence on the proportions and shape of the orbit, and the bones that constitute it. In the brachycephalic group for instance, the lacrimal bone does not reach the orbital margin, but leaves an edge of the maxilla in the position it would otherwise occupy.

8:2   Ordinarily six bones form the dog's orbit; the frontal, lacrimal, sphenoid, palatine, zygomatic and maxillary (Fig. 125). But the last bone only encroaches into the orbital region to a small extent in the extreme anteroventral region, and even then it is well external to the periorbita and true orbit.

8:3   On the frontal bone, there is a rudimentary process called the zygomatic process, and on the zygomatic bone below it, there is another prominence called the frontal process. These

two are joined by a bridge of fibrous tissue containing a few bands of smooth muscle, called the *orbital ligament*. This ligament alone completes the lateral closure of the orbit, which otherwise merges into the temporal fossa.

8:4   The size of the dog or of the dog's head has little relationship to the size of its orbit, an important detail to know when planning surgery of the extraocular muscles or an enucleation. A large headed dog may have a larger eye than a smaller breed, but the orbit may not necessarily increase in diameter to an equal extent.

8:5   The contents of the orbit consists of the eyeball and optic nerve, the extraocular muscles, the lacrimal gland, blood vessels and nerves; the spaces between these are filled with fat and fasciae. The contents are wholly enclosed within a conical fibrous *periorbital* membrane.

147

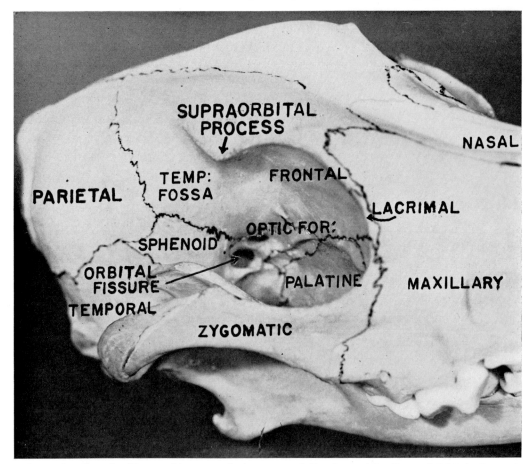

Fig. 125.   The orbital bones. (Prince, et al. *Anatomy and Histology of the Eye and Orbit in Domestic Animals,* courtesy of Charles C Thomas.)

8:6   The various orbital foramina through which the orbital nerves and blood vessels pass, differ considerably in size and shape. The *optic foramen* is the pathway for the second or optic nerve and the internal ophthalmic artery.

8:7   The *orbital fissure,* separated from the optic foramen by a bridge of bone about 1 mm wide, is the largest of three adjacent foramina. It carries the third, fourth, and sixth nerves, the ophthalmic division of the fifth nerve, and the orbital vein.

8:8   Because the dog does not pos-

sess a complete bony orbit, there are several nerve trunks, which although they do not serve the orbit in any way, are only separated from its contents by the thin periorbita. This close apposition means they are in a surgically vulnerable position. The sphenopalatine nerve, the sphenopalatine ganglion, infraorbital nerve, sphenopalatine artery, infraorbital artery, deep facial nerve, and zygomatic gland (Par. 8:9) are those structures which have to be carefully considered in this respect.

8:9   In addition to the lacrimal and nictitans glands which are common to all of the animals, the dog has a *zygomatic gland* situated in the orbital region. In most animals the dorsal and ventral buccal glands extend along the cheek. In the dog the dorsal buccal gland lies inferior and lateral to the orbit, against the internal surface of the anterior portion of the zygomatic arch. For this reason it is referred to as the zygomatic gland although its salivary secretions pass through the ducts to empty into the mouth near the last upper molar tooth.

8:10   The *lacrimal gland* lies within the periorbita, is well demarcated and is shaped like the tip of a spatula. Its long axis is directly against the orbital ligament and almost symmetrically situated anteriorly and posteriorly from it. The dorsal end is just below the tip of the zygomatic process of the frontal bone and further down it has a tendinous anchorage to the frontal process of the zygomatic bone. It has an appearance very similar to muscle. From fifteen to twenty small ducts open from it into the conjunctival sac at the superior fornix where they are not easily seen. The lacrimal gland usually has a maximum width of 12.5 mm, a depth (dorsoventral) of 15 mm, and is fairly flat.

Diseases[2, 3]

8:11   Affections of the orbit include: (1) congenital anomalies, (2) displacement of the eyeball (*i.e.* exophthalmos, enophthalmos), (3) cellulitis and periostitis, (4) tumors, and (5) injuries.

8:12   *Congenital anomalies* of the eyeball include, (1) anophthalmos, (2) microphthalmos, and (3) congenital glaucoma. *Anophthalmos* (Fig. 126) is rare. The globe is replaced by a small solid or cystic mass. In *microphthalmos*, the eyeball is diminished in size in all diameters. This condition cannot be considered rare, may occur in any breed, but more recently has been observed in the poodle, miniature schnauzer and collie breeds. The eyeball may be functional or an associated congenital cataract or detached retina may be present. Barone and Lescure[4] consider this phenomenon as a deficiency in the ocular edification with a hereditary aspect. *Congenital glaucoma* (Par. 9:37) results in an enlarged eyeball (buphthalmos, hydrophthalmos). I have encountered but one case, in a cocker spaniel puppy.

8:13   *Displacement of the eyeball.* The most important signs of diseases of the orbit are *exophthalmos* (proptosis or protrusion of the eyeball from the orbit), and *enophthalmos* (recession of the eyeball into the orbit). As compared to the human there are, of course, many variations of the normal in the dog. Some eyes are naturally recessed, *e.g.* the collie breed, while others naturally protrude, *e.g.* pekingese, pugs, Boston terriers. It is, therefore, important to compare one eye with the other in the same animal, observing the eyes from every aspect (Par. 2:15).

Exophthalmos

8:14   Exophthalmos is a common sign in affections of the orbit. The globe often appears to be larger or glaucomatous but it is the widening of the palpebral fissure that produces this illusion. There is rarely an increase in tension. In fact, the eye may well have a tension lower than its fellow eye. Exophthalmos is usually unilateral.

8:15   There are four conditions of the orbit and periorbital structures in which varying degrees of exophthalmos

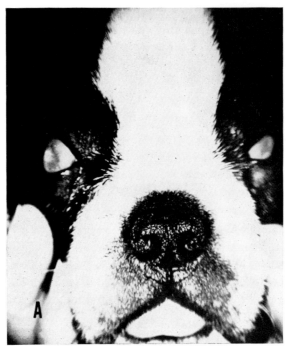

A

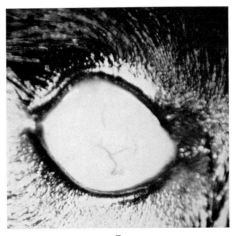

B

Fig. 126.   *A*. Bilateral anophthalmos. *B*. Close up of one side.

are exhibited. It is quite possible to confuse these and arrive at a hasty and incorrect diagnosis. Since the treatment for each differs greatly and the dogs life may well depend upon the correct diagnosis and proper treatment, it becomes imperative that exophthalmos not be considered lightly.

8:16   1. *Lid abscesses.* (Fig. 59A) Infection of the lid (Par. 4:71) causes but a moderate degree of exophthalmos but the swelling is fluctuating and painful. This condition must be distinguished from a true orbital cellulitis (retrobulbar abscess). Treatment of lid abscesses consists of surgical drainage, curettage, and the instillation of an antibiotic (Par. 4:71).

8:17 2. *Orbital Cellulitis* (retrobulbar abscess) (Plate 8A) Exophthalmos is a prominent symptom when an abscess develops in the retrobulbar area. In addition, there is swelling of the lids, hypertrophy and protrusion of the membrane nictitans, chemosis, impairment of mobility of the eyeball, subjective pain when pressure is applied, and often the dog will exhibit extreme pain when an attempt is made to open its mouth. The cause of orbital cellulitis is obscure but several factors must be considered. Awns have a way of working up through the mouth into the retrobulbar area, hookworm larvae migration is believed to be responsible on occasion, extension of disease of the nasal accessory sinuses may be a factor, and, involvement of the unusual zygomatic gland of the dog (Par. 8:9) cannot be discounted.

8:18 *Treatment* of retrobulbar abscesses consists of surgical drainage behind the last upper molar on the affected side, local instillation and systemic administration of penicillin.

Technique.

(1) General anesthesia and insert mouth speculum.
(2) Palpate soft area posterior to the last upper molar. There is often a red, raised area evident.
(3) Incise with No. 11 Bard Parker blade.
(4) Insert smooth probe to retrobulbar area (Fig. 127). Pus may follow its withdrawal. Enlarge opening by spread-

ings tips of long hemostatic forceps.
(5) Irrigate gently with antiseptic solution or hydrogen peroxide. A teat canula and 5-cc hypodermic syringe is useful for this purpose. Collect irrigation material in gauze or cotton held in mouth.
(6) Instill 500,000 units of penicillin G (crystalline-potassium) into incision site and towards retrobulbar area with 2 inch, 22 gauge needle.
(7) Intramuscular injection of long acting penicillin.

8:19 Sometimes the abscess has not organized and little to no pus will follow the incision and probing. Usually, however, an appreciable drainage will follow. In either event there is noticeable improvement within twenty-four hours and complete recovery within several days to a week. The exophthalmos, membrane nictitans protrusion, and lid and conjunctival swellings subside quickly. It may be necessary to administer systemic penicillin more than once or to even re-establish drainage of the surgical site in the severely involved cases.

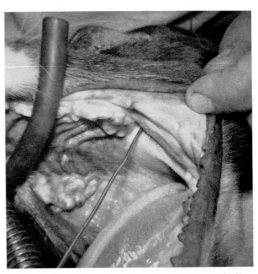

Fig. 127. Direction of probe to left retrobulbar area.

8:20   3. *Eosinophilic Myositis* (Plate 8B). This is a less common, but strikingly similar disease to orbital cellulitis in many respects. Whereas the symptoms are quite alike, this disease causes death in many instances. The blood picture reveals a substantial increase in the eosinophil count and the disease presents a characteristic clinical picture. There is symmetrical swelling of the masseter, temporalis, and pterygoid muscles. Like in orbital cellulitis, there is a variable degree of exophthalmos, edema of the lids, hypertrophy and protrusion of the membrane nictitans, and the mouth may be held open slightly. According to Winter and Stephenson,[5] the enlarged pterygoid and temporalis muscles press on the retrobulbar tissue and cause the exophthalmos.

8:21   From our observations and those of others, there are clearly differences in the manifestations of eosinophilic myositis. Great importance has been placed by some on eosinophil levels, with an increase of between 12 and 20 per cent thought to be significant. Yet, Harding and Owen[6] examined the blood of 50 German shepherd dogs which had never suffered from eosinophilic myositis and found 11 with eosinophil levels between 10 and 28 per cent. They believe a blood examination might prove deceptive. Their cases included six German shepherds and one Bedlington terrier. During attacks it was possible to open the jaws to their full extent, although it appeared to cause pain.

8:22   We have encountered the disease in both the German shepherds and Weimariner breeds. Aside from the increase in eosinophil count, we have noted that in the acute, severe cases it became *impossible* to open the jaws to their fullest extent, even when the ani-

mal was placed under deep general anesthesia. This, of course, would not be true in a case of orbital cellulitis.

8:23   Attacks of eosinophilic myositis last from ten to twenty-one days. Spontaneous recovery may occur or the animal may well succumb without proper treatment. One or both eyes may be involved, regardless of whether the attack is mild or severe.

8:24   *Treatment.* Thus far, no factors which might have initiated attacks of eosinophilic myositis have been discovered. It would appear unlikely that an infectious agent is responsible. Antibiotics have proven useless. It is difficult to assess the efficacy of therapeutic measures since so little has been published on the subject. However, in recent years the systemic use of the steroids has proven to be specific in those cases which I have seen, and ACTH was found to be a promising therapeutic agent by Harding and Owen.[6] In recovered cases, one can expect wasting of the temporalis and masseter muscles. Atrophy of the postorbital fat can, in turn, create an enophthalmos (Fig. 8D).

8:25   4. *Retrobulbar tumors.* Neoplasms of the orbit in man, although not considered rare, are still not so common that single institutions can collect a large series. The same can be said for cases occurring in the dog. Smythe[7] mentions osteosarcoma of the orbit causing exophthalmos and eventual blindness. Williams et al.[8] reported that a retrobulbar glioma of the optic nerve developed along the course of the left optic nerve to the optic nerve to the optic chiasm and then along the course of the right optic nerve.

8:26   The following text is in summary of my series.[9] Each of the retrobulbar tumor cases in this series (7) exhibited one or all of the following, depending on the stage of development:

1. exophthalmos, globe deviation, diminished movement;
2. swellings around the globe;
3. prominent, hypertrophied membrane nictitans;
4. pupil dilated and/or eccentric;
5. exposure keratitis;
6. blindness.

8:27 Age range was from four to eleven and six breeds were represented. Tumors included neurogenic sarcoma, chondrosarcoma, squamous cell carcinoma, meningioma, adenocarcinoma of salivary gland origin, and a rhabdomyosarcoma. The seventh did not come to necropsy. All were unilateral except one (squamous cell carcinoma) (Fig. 128). A Boxer with the rhabdomyosarcoma (Plate 8E) presented a very prominent papilledema (Par. 11:86) along with the early exophthalmos. This type tumor is considered rare in man.

8:28 Most of the cases had a prior diagnosis of glaucoma when I first saw them, yet, the intraocular tension was normal or below in each instance. Exophthalmos is not part of the glaucoma complex. A diagnosis of retrobulbar tumor is relatively easy to arrive at and is based on the history and *gradual* onset of the exophthalmos.

8:29 Exploratory surgery was performed in two cases. One was immediately euthanized on learning of the hopelessness of the situation. The second dog was euthanized four months following surgery when it was evident that regrowth and further extension was in progress. Whereas surgery for removal of a postorbital tumor with preservation of the globe is possible (Kroenlein technique), most often exenteration

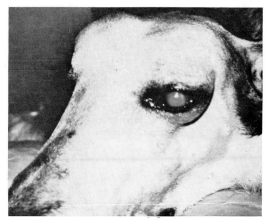

Fig. 128. Bilateral, retrobulbar squamous cell carcinoma. Note swellings above and around the eyes.

of the orbit (Par. 8:42) will be necessary to insure patient comfort or prevent metastasis when a primary involvement is suspected.

Enophthalmos (Plate 8D)

8:30 Enophthalmos is an uncommon sign in affections of the orbit. The eye appears smaller but is not necessarily. It is the narrowing of the palpebral fissure and recession of the globe that effects this appearance.

8:31 *Causes.* While not as common as exophthalmos, there are a number of possible causes for enophthalmos. Following trauma or surgery of the orbit, the postorbital fat may absorb, thus allowing the eye to sink back. A hematoma of the orbit may encapsulate, slowly absorb and then result in an enophthalmos. Cicatricial contraction following orbital injuries and cellulitis may cause a recession of the eyeball.

8:32 Enophthalmos is a distinct possibility in the dog recovered from eosinophilic myositis (Par. 8:20) due to the atrophy of the surrounding muscles and postorbital fat. Phthisis bulbi (Par. 7:55) (Plate 8C), a shrunken fibrotic globe as a sequela to endophthalmitis, invariably produces an enophthalmos.

8:33 Reduction in size of the eyeball due to congenital microphthalmos (Par. 8:12) is another cause, and anophthalmos, in which the eyeball is but a small solid cystic mass (Par. 8:12) (Fig. 126), is still another.

8:34 The possible effects of enophthalmos include (1) epiphora (excess tearing) because the puncti are no longer in the proper position to drain the tears; (2) mucous accumulation in the lower conjunctival cul-de-sac; (3) some alteration in overall vision because of the muscle imbalance which occurs; and, (4) corneal drying because the lids are not in approximation with, and thus able to wipe the cornea.

Operations and Procedures Involving the Eye and the Orbit

Enucleation

8:35 *Indications* for enucleation include (1) the presence of suppurative panophthalmitis following foreign body penetration or disease process; (2) irreplaceable and/or gangrenous luxated eyeball with nerve and vessel rupture; (3) severe irreparable injuries in which the form of the eyeball cannot be preserved; (4) pain in a blind eye which cannot be relieved by less radical means; (5) massive anterior staphyloma, if the eye is blind, troublesome, and disfiguring (for cosmetic improvement); (6) the occurrence of chronic conjunctivitis, corneal, or eyelid disease due to an acquired phthisis bulbi or congenital microphthalmia; and, (7) the presence of an intraocular or retrobulbar malignant neoplasm not amendable to surgery or radiation therapy.

8:36 In the practice of veterinary medicine, many enucleations have been and are being performed unnecessarily. Enucleation is selected as the procedure of choice in several conditions which will respond beautifully to the proper medical or surgical procedure. In addition, enucleation is often the consequence of a poorly conceived and executed line of treatment. The one-eyed dog is often a long living example of some veterinarian's apathy or inability to cope with an ofttimes simple ocular problem. In most instances, prolapse of the iris as the result of injury or ulcer, badly ulcerated eyes, scarred and pigmented corneas, luxated globes, and glaucoma are *not* indications for enucleation.

8:37 *Technique.* A true enucleation is performed by removing the eyeball from Tenon's capsule and the bulbar conjunctiva, leaving the extraocular muscles and soft parts of the orbit intact. This procedure (subconjunctival ablation) is preferable to the commonly practiced near exenteration (Par. 8:42) in which conjunctiva, muscles and adjacent structures are removed. By preserving these tissues a better cosmetic

---

Plate 8.

    A. Retrobulbar abscess. Note conjunctival chemosis and exophthalmos.

    B. Eosinophilic myositis. Note protrusion and drying of the membrane nictitans associated with the exophthalmos.

    C. Phthisis bulbi. Enophthalmic globe held out with forceps.

    D. Enophthalmos. Left eye. Note distance from medial canthus to the globe.

    E. Retrobulbar rhabdomyosarcoma. Right orbit. Note exophthalmos and exposure keratitis. Courtesy: Dr. Raymond Sytek, Rockford, Illinois.

    F. Retrobulbar osteoma. Right orbit. Note exophthalmos and the superior, lateral deviation of the globe.

Plate 8

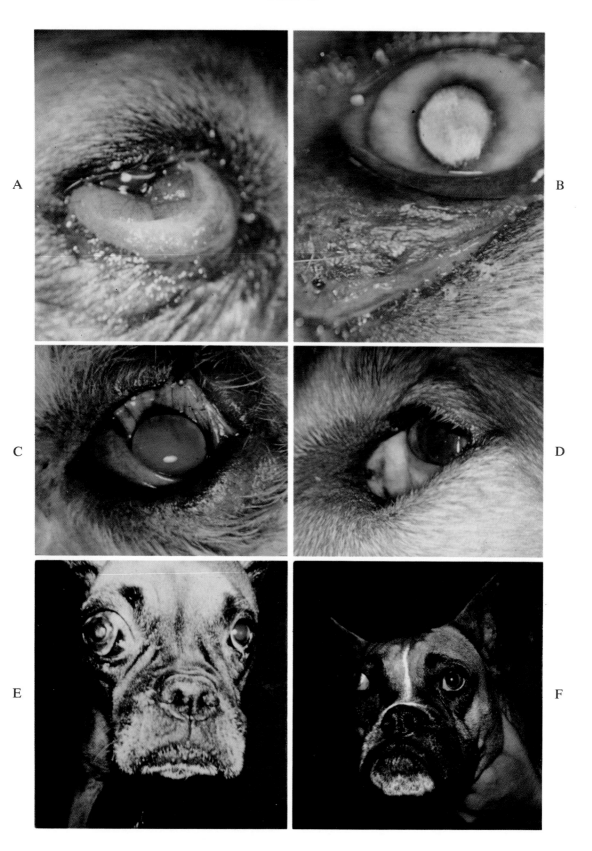

result is achieved since there is far less depression following final healing. In addition, this technique offers the advantage of preparing the socket for the insertion of an implant within the conjunctiva and Tenon's capsule, with still less depression resulting, or, for the use of an implant and prosthesis or artificial eye (Par. 8:47).

8:38 *Steps:*

1. The eye is proptosed (Par. 6:137), if this is possible. A canthotomy (Par. 4:12) (Fig. 40) will facilitate the performance of this step. An incision is made near the limbus through the conjunctiva and Tenon's capsule down to the sclera. The released structures are either, (*a*) grasped in the four quadrants with small Allis forceps, or, (*b*) held away from the globe by sutures, or, (*c*) a purse string suture of 4–0 chromic catgut can be loosely placed near the edge.

2. The conjunctiva and Tenon's capsule are undermined with tenotomy scissors, severing the extraocular muscle attachments as the undermining proceeds to the posterior part of the globe.

3. With the globe exposed and the conjunctiva reflected away, a regular tonsil snare, or, preferably one operated from an electrocautery unit, is used to encircle the globe and to sever the optic nerve and accompanying vessels.

4. The eyeball is removed and the edges of the conjunctiva and Tenon's capsule are drawn together with either the previously placed purse string suture or by using post placed interrupted catgut sutures. If an implant is to be used, it is placed in this socket before the sutures are drawn up.

5. The membrane nictitans and its gland is then severed at its base and removed.

6. Approximately ¼ inch of the margins of the lids are removed and the wound edges apposed with the suture material of choice.

8:39 The wound may be bandaged in the conventional manner described (Par. 3:81) or by placing a stent bandage. Ordinarily there is little hemorrhage or serum accumulation attending this procedure, especially when the electrocautery tonsil snare is used. If a prosthesis is to be used (Par. 8:44), the membrane nictitans is left intact and the lid margins, of course, are not cut or sutured.

Evisceration

8:40 This operation differs from enucleation in that, in evisceration the cornea and entire contents of the eyeball are removed, but the sclera is left intact. The only indication for this procedure is in those instances in which an intrascleral implant is to be used as an artificial eye (Par. 8:46), or to provide a stump to lend mobility to an externally placed prosthesis (Par. 8:47).

8:41 The operation is contraindicated in malignant tumors of either the eye or retrobulbar area, in shrunken eyeballs, or when a generalized panophthalmitis with a weak, ectatic sclera is present.

Exenteration

8:42 Exenteration of the orbit includes removal of the globe, conjunctiva, extraocular muscles, and surrounding structures within the orbit. The only indication for this radical procedure is in certain cases of malignancy, *i.e.*, retrobulbar neoplasia or extention of a uveal tract tumor into the orbit itself. Loppnow and Link[10] describe a case in which a malignant melanoma of the iris and ciliary body necessitated enucleation. Several months later the orbital cavity was found to be involved. On a subsequent necropsy, metastases to the lungs, heart muscle, and kidneys was disclosed.

8:43   Following exenteration of the orbit the closed lids and skin retract into the orbit with disfigurement, but the patient's life may well be saved by virtue of this procedure (Par. 8:29). Cosmetic improvement may be attained by burying various silicone and inert plastic preparations manufactured for that purpose.

Artificial Eyes

8:44   Eye prostheses have seldom been used in the dog despite the fact that prosthetic devices to stimulate the enucleated eye were developed and used as long ago as the latter part of the nineteenth century. The operation has never become standard procedure in the dog because of economic factors, the nuisance of maintaining the devices, and a high percentage of failures. Two types of artificial eyes may be used: (1) The permanent intrascleral implant; and, (2) the shell-shaped prosthesis in common use by human subjects follow-

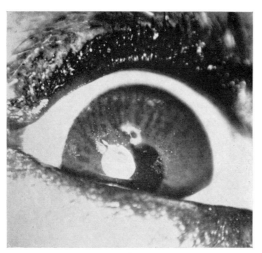

Fig. 129. The shell-shaped human prosthesis adapted for use in the dog.

ing enucleation. This type is removed and re-inserted daily for cleansing purposes.

8:45   Simpson[11] reported success in the prosthetic reconstruction of the canine globe by the implantation of an intrascleral prosthesis, following evisceration of the globe (Par. 8:40). In order to insure success in a majority of the cases, however, he found that an exacting technique was necessary. Also, that a chronic conjunctivitis resulting from the implant required supervision by the owner or else separation would occur and the implant would extrude.

8:46   Keil[12] describes the use of a plastic intrascleral implant which is held in place by a stainless steel purse string suture. I have had repeated failures using this procedure. In each instance extrusion took place several weeks following surgery or the implant was "pawed out" by the patient. Evisceration and the use of an intrascleral implant is, theoretically, the procedure of choice. However, since the sclera has no blood supply, it often will not heal to the implant. In addition, the "foreign body reaction" predisposes to extrusion.

8:47   The externally placed, shell-shaped prosthesis used in the human subject can be used successfully in the dog as well (Fig. 129). Following enucleation (Par. 8:37) a ball of either glass, plastic or silicone intended for this purpose is inserted in the cavity and the edges of the conjunctiva and Tenon's capsule are drawn together over the implant. The membrane nictitans and lid margins are left intact.

8:48   A "conformer" is then placed underneath the lids and the membrane nictitans and the area bandaged in the conventional manner (Par. 3:81) (Fig. 31). Dressings are changed at two- to three-day intervals with removal, cleansing, and replacing of the conformer at each dressing. After approximately three weeks the cavity has healed sufficiently to allow fitting of the "glass eye." A regular "stock" prosthesis may be used, but to insure a good fit and matching eye a custom-made shell is preferable.

8:49 When placed underneath the lids, with the membrane nictitans serving as an additional aid to its retention, the average dog tolerates this type prosthesis quite well. However, as is the case in the human, the "eye" should be removed at least once a day for the purpose of cleansing the cavity and the prosthesis. Needless to say, the average owner is reluctant to assume the expense and bother associated with this type of surgical procedure.

8:50 Regardless of the type of implant used, their successful use depends upon the observance of (1) complete asepsis in the operative procedure; (2) incising the conjunctiva and Tenon's capsule close to the limbus; (3) control of bleeding before the implant is inserted; and, (4) placing the implant within Tenon's capsule as well as the conjunctiva, with the closure of these membranes over the implant made without undue tension.

Luxation of the Globe

8:51 Luxation or proptosing of the eyeball occurs most frequently in the brachycephalic breeds as a result of automobile injuries or encounters with larger dogs. Shortly after luxation the eyeball becomes inflamed and congested and the chemotic conjunctiva protrudes beyond the lid margins. Since the lids cannot close properly over the proptosed globe, corneal desiccation occurs. A subconjunctival hemorrhage may be present as the result of a tooth puncture. In severe cases a retrobulbar hemorrhage is usually present.

8:52 *Treatment.* The treatment and prognosis is largely dependent upon the degree of damage to the extraocular muscles and to the blood and nerve supply to the eye. It is usually difficult to ascertain the extent of vessel and nerve injury at the time of the accident. The first consideration should always be to replace the globe as quickly as possible. Permanent damage, requiring enucleation, will be evident within several days.

8:53 In simple and very recent cases of luxation, replacement of the globe is easily accomplished following simple cleansing and lubrication with an antibiotic ointment. Under short acting anesthesia, the lids are elevated with forceps or lid retractors, a pad of wet cotton is applied to the globe, and moderate pressure is applied with the fingers. If the eyeball "snaps back" into the orbit with no tendency to protrude, no further treatment is needed.

8:54 In the more complicated cases, and in those instances in which the globe has been luxated for several hours or a day, the following routine has been used with considerable success.

8:55 *Procedure:*
(1) *Canthotomy.* (Par. 4:11) (Fig. 40). Elongation of the palpebral fissure not only facilitates replacement of the globe, but failure to perform this initial step may make it impossible to do so.
(2) *Retrobulbar steroid injection* (Par. 9:98) (Fig. 133). A systemic dose of a steroid placed in the retrobulbar area aids greatly in reducing the edema and dissipating the hemorrhage back of and surrounding the globe. This, in turn, enables the eyeball to "settle back" into its proper position in the orbit in a mat-

ter of days instead of a week or more. Penicillin G (crystalline-potassium) may be added to the injection. The use of intravenous mannitol as an effective ocular hypotensive agent with a quite acceptable margin of safety shows promise of also being helpful.

(3) *Lid suture placement* (Fig. 139). Three mattress sutures are placed through the skin opposite the lid margins at the medial (nasal), lateral (temporal) and center positions. These are left untied until the globe is replaced.

(4) *Replacement of the globe.* The eyeball is returned to the orbit in the manner described (Par. 8:53). If this becomes impossible because of the retrobulbar swelling, the lids and lid margins are carefully worked into position over the proptosed globe and the sutures are brought into place and tied. The canthotomy incision is closed with one or more interrupted sutures in the usual manner. By completely covering the eye in this manner, it remains protected until the postorbital swelling is reduced and it can assume its normal position in the orbit. A drop of atropine and an antibiotic preparation are instilled prior to the final closure.

8:56   *Aftercare.* Usually in forty-eight hours the swelling has reduced to the degree that either a lateral or medial suture can be removed. This enables the clinician to "take a peek" at the cornea, ascertain globe viability, and as to whether the eye is "saved" or must now be enucleated. As the swelling recedes a second peripheral suture may be removed. Finally, when it appears that the globe will be protected by the natural opening and closing of the lids, the center suture is removed.

8:57   In some instances the globe is deviated because of tearing of the extraocular muscle attachments. This deviation is usually to the temporal side and,

unless it is severe, the eyeball most often straightens itself in time. When considerable muscle damage and deviation is noted at the time of the luxation, it is best to attempt correction along with replacement. This entails undermining the bulbar conjunctiva on the nasal side, finding the torn muscle ends and bringing them together. When this becomes impossible to do, an inverted mattress suture of stainless steel or plastic is placed in the deep episcleral tissue near the limbus on the nasal side, is brought through the membrane nictitans, and is tied over a button or pad in the nasal fold. This suture is allowed to remain for a week or more.

References

1. Prince, Jack H., Diesem, Charles D., Eglitis, Irma and Ruskell, Gordon L.: *Anatomy and Histology of the Eye and Orbit in Domestic Animals,* Springfield, Charles C Thomas, p. 65–71, 1960.
2. Magrane, William G.: *Diseases of the Orbit,* Vet. Med., 449–451, 1957.
3. *Canine Medicine,* 2nd ed., Santa Barbara, American Veterinary Publications, Inc., p. 528–530, 1959.
4. Barone, R. and Lescure, F.: Hétérochromie et Microphtalmie, chez le Chien, Extrait de la Revue de Médecine Vétérinaire, *110,* 769, 1959.
5. Winter, Hans, and Stephenson, H. C.: A Case of Eosinophilic Myositis in a Dog, Cornell Vet., *42,* p. 531, 1952.
6. Harding, H. P., and Owen, L. N.: Eosinophilic Myositis in the Dog, Jour. Comp. Path. & Therap., *66,* p. 109, 1956.
7. Smythe, R. H.: *Veterinary Ophthalmology,* London, Bailliere Tindall & Cox, p. 163, 1956.
8. Williams, J. O., Garlick, E. C., Beard, D. C.: Glioma of the Optic Nerve of a Dog, J.A.V.M.A., *138,* 377–378, 1961.
9. Magrane, William G.: Tumors of the Eye and Orbit in the Dog, Proceedings XVIIth World Veterinary Congress, Hanover, Germany, *2,* p. 1095–1098, 1963.
10. Loppnaw, H. and Link, E.: Berl. U. Münch Tierärzt. Wschr., *174*(16), 317–321, 1961.
11. Simpson, H. D.: Reconstructive Surgery of the Canine Eye, No. Am. Vet., 37, 1060–1065, 1956.
12. Keil, John H., Jr.: Mobile Ocular Prosthesis, Jen-Sal Small Animal Topics, *1* #3, 21–24, 1959.

Chapter 9

GLAUCOMA

9:1 The reader may be somewhat surprised to see that an entire chapter is devoted to glaucoma when, as a specific entity, it occurs with comparative infrequency. I am of the belief that glaucoma is the leading cause of blindness in the middle aged dog. Since glaucoma is an emergency type disease, with irreversible blindness ensuing within hours to several days, it becomes extremely important that the veterinary clinician understand this condition. Accuracy in diagnosis, classification, and knowledge of the proper medical or surgical procedures to fit the classification will save or prevent loss of vision. For this reason, the importance of a disease cannot be overemphasized.

Anatomy and Physiology

9:2 Certain parts of the eye are particularly important in any consideration of the physiologic mechanisms, the pathology, and the medical and surgical treatment of the glaucomas. These structures are in the anterior segment of the globe (Fig. 120) and include the iris and ciliary body, the anterior and posterior chambers, the filtration angle, and the intrascleral drainage plexus (Fig. 121).

9:3 The iris divides the aqueous cavity into an *anterior* and *posterior* chamber. The ciliary body, via its ciliary processes, secretes the *aqueous humor* (Par. 7:8). The aqueous humor fills the anterior and posterior chambers and drains through the filtration angle into the intrascleral plexus (Fig. 130).

9:4 The filtration angle (angle of the iris) is a circular recess where cornea, sclera, the ciliary border of the iris and the ciliary body meet. In the angle a peculiar framework of *trabeculae* with irregular spaces (spaces of Fontana) are found. The trabeculum is also called the *pectinate ligament* of the iris. Troncoso[1] describes the trabeculum of the dog as being in contact with a well-developed venous plexus known as the intrascleral vascular plexus (*plexus venosus sclerae*). This plexus is formed by a thick network of large interlacing veins lodged in large canals inside the scleral wall.

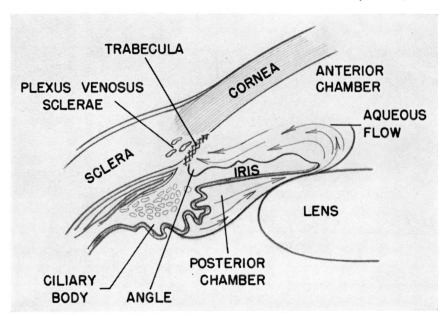

Fig. 130.   Mode of aqueous production and flow from the posterior to the anterior chamber and thence to the drainage angle.

Its superficial branches spread over the inner scleral surface and are in contact with or run between the trabeculum fibers. They are called trabecular veins and it is through them that the aqueous filling the sinus is absorbed by the blood. These vessels function in a manner similar to the canal of Schlemm in man.

9:5   Considerable research has been conducted in aqueous drainage in the dog. The existence of the continual current of aqueous from the anterior chamber into the episcleral vessels was postulated by Leber,[2] mainly by experimental work in animals. Friedenwald and Pierce,[3] working with a modified Leber manometer, have shown by experiments that in dogs there is a constant current of liquid from the chamber into the episcleral veins. They also showed experimentally that other ocular tissues, especially the iris, take part in the elimination of the aqueous. Intraocular

tension tends to lower when the iris is under vasodilatation as in acute iritis (Par. 7:34), and when the cornea is irritated.

Methods of Diagnosis[4]

9:6   Glaucoma, whether it be in man or animals, is not, in itself, a disease entity. Instead, it consists of a variety group of conditions which have as their common feature an abnormal elevation of intraocular pressure. This group may be referred to as the glaucomas.

9:7   Normal intraocular pressure is that which is compatible with the continued health and function of the eye. In the dog, however, we must give more emphasis to statistical averages in our computation of normal pressures because of our inability to perform perimetry and other exact visual function tests.

9:8   A distinction has been made between the use of the terms "pressure" and "tension" in relation to the eye. The term "intraocular pressure" refers to the pressure of the intraocular fluid within the eye which can only be measured by means of a manometer. The "tension" of the eye is a measure of the state of tension of its tunics, being estimated either digitally or by means of a tonometer. In addition to intraocular pressure, tension depends upon the thickness and rigidity of the tunics, the surface area, and probably other factors.

9:9 Manometry is not practical for use in clinical veterinary ophthalmology, whereas digital palpation and tonometry are. In this discussion of canine glaucoma, then, the term "tension" will be used to denote rise and fall of intraocular pressure.

Tonometry

9:10 Tonometry is defined as the measurement of the impressibility of the tunics of the eye by deforming forces applied to these tunics. The impressibility depends on the resistance of the eyeball which, in turn, depends on the intraocular pressure. Thus, tonometry gives a measure, however approximate, of the intraocular pressure.

9:11 In digital tonometry (Par. 2: 29) (Fig. 20), the two index fingers are placed upon the dog's upper lid. By alternating pressure on the globe from one finger tip to the other, pressing more downward than backward, one can get some idea of the degree of tension by comparison with the other eye, if normal, or with a healthy eye of another dog. By way of comparison, a glaucomatous eye will feel like a hard apple, while an eye with normal tension will feel approximately like a soft gelatin worm capsule. Digital tonometry is especially useful when the intraocular tension is either quite low or quite high,

and should be the means of measurement employed when the corneal epithelium is abnormal or eroded, or when a refractory dog is examined.

9:12 Instrumental tonometry, by far the more accurate means of measuring intraocular tension, should be used when possible (Par. 2:32) (Fig. 22). The tonometer, by movement of a needle upon a scale, records resistance offered to definite weights used to produce an indentation of the cornea. Readings as low as 16 and as high as 30 mm Hg may be considered within the normal range in the dog (Par. 2:33).

9:13 In cooperative animals, readings can be made following two instillations, separated by a five-minute interval, of topical anesthetics.

9:14 The dog should be placed on a table in a sitting position. An assistant, or the owner, restrains the animal's head in such manner that the eyes are directed upward, the lids are separated, and the tonometer is allowed to rest by its own weight upon the center of the upturned cornea. In the separation of the lids, undue pressure must not be exerted on the eyeball itself, thus influencing the reading. The nictitating membrane often proves a deterent to the accurate placement of the footplate of the tonometer and many readings will, of necessity, be taken with the footplate between the center and upper limbal area. The degree of accuracy achieved in man with the use of the tonometer cannot always be attained in the dog but, with patience, a good approximation of tension is almost always attainable. An instillation of a suitable ophthalmic antiseptic or antibiotic preparation to the tested eye is indicated, following the procedure, to forestall a possible infection from the footplate or from its abrasive action on the cornea. The tonometer itself must be cared for as a delicate instrument, including cleaning following each use if it is expected to give consistent and accurate readings.

9:15   Lovekin[5] suggests that intraocular tension be measured by rolling the dog over on his back, with his nose in the air pointing slightly to the left to take the tension of the right eye, and then slightly to the right to take the tension of the left eye. The nictitating membrane should be held gently out of the way, and the tonometer placed vertically on the center of the cornea in order to achieve the most accuracy. She[5] found the highest normal intraocular pressure to be 26 mm Hg in her series.

Clinical Signs

9:16   The diagnosis of glaucoma in the dog is relatively simple since the animal is usually presented for an examination only when the clinical signs are exaggerated and visible to the owner. Important early signs of pain and of disturbance of vision go unnoticed and, undoubtedly, in many instances the dog has been subjected to transient attacks of pressure increases before a final and permanent increase manifests itself. Whereas this simplifies diagnosis, it makes adequate treatment more difficult—especially as regards the preservation of vision. Too many animals have reached the absolute (blind) stage before being examined.

Characteristics of Glaucoma

9:17   There are many general characteristics of glaucoma, all of which, of course, are not exhibited in any one animal. A great deal depends upon the nature of the attack, and whether it falls into a primary or secondary classification. The general characteristics include;

(1) increase in intraocular tension; (2) pain; (3) cloudy, "steamy" cornea; (4) insensitive cornea; (5) shallow anterior chamber; (6) dilatation of pupil, with no response to light; (7) episcleral vascularization (congestion of episcleral vessels); (8) loss of vision (partial or complete); (9) buphthalmos (hydrophthalmos); (10) cupping of the optic disc; (11) atrophy of the optic disc and retina; and (12) atrophy of the iris.

9:18   *Increase in intraocular tension* has been discussed under tonometry.

9:19   *Pain.* Pain is produced by pressure and pull on the ciliary nerves in the eye. In obtaining case histories, some owners will volunteer the information that the dog has exhibited pain, which is often displayed by the animal rubbing the eye on the rug, against the owner's leg, or on furniture. Upon digital palpation, many dogs will wince; others appear to suffer little or no pain. Pain seems to depend somewhat upon the duration of the attack—the longer the period of increased tension, the less pain—but some dogs evidence little or no pain at any time. However, after having an increased tension for a year or more, some dogs change completely in disposition and become extremely refractory. When the tension is relieved, they usually again become docile—a gratifying aftermath.

9:20   *Cloudy, "Steamy" Cornea.* This is manifested most prominently in acute congestive glaucoma, less so in the chronic and absolute stages. The cloudiness has been attributed to an edema of the substantia propria and a collection of fluid under and between the epithelial cells.

9:21   When tension is decreased by medical or surgical means, the cornea quickly clears unless the eye has been under extreme pressure for a long period. In some dogs, the fundic detail is revealed on ophthalmoscopic examination; in others, because of the cloudy media, this is not possible. In several instances, increased tension over a long period has resulted in a striate keratitis. Rucks in Descemet's membrane, due to edema and swelling of the substantia propria, causes finger-like processes or streaks in the cornea. These opacities tend to remain permanently, even after the tension has been rendered normal by surgery.

9:22 *Insensitive Cornea.* Increased tension may cause the cornea to become insensitive from pressure upon nerve filaments. In the dog, when a glaucomatous eye is brushed with a feather or wisp of cotton, there will be no reflex blinking as in the normal eye (Par. 2:20).

9:23 *Shallow Anterior Chamber.* In acute congestive glaucoma, the anterior chamber is often shallow (Par. 2:24), due to the anterior displacement of the iris and lens. The cause of this is probably an increase in volume or swelling of the vitreous body, accompanied by an edema and swelling of the ciliary processes. The chamber depth in the dog can be approximated, and compared with the normal eye, by observing the eye from the lateral aspect with pen-light and binocular loupe. When the observer's eye becomes "practiced" to depth perception, shallow chambers can readily be seen when viewing the eye from the front. Whereas a shallow anterior chamber is usually associated with primary acute attacks of glaucoma, it may be observed in instances of secondary glaucoma, *e.g.*, types of lens subluxation, swelling of the lens in cataract formation (Par. 10:36), and in iris *bombé* (Par. 7:37).

9:24 *Dilatation of the Pupil* (Plate 9A). Probably the most constant and significant clinical sign of glaucoma in the dog is full dilatation of the pupil with no response to light stimuli (Par. 7:17). This is also a constant finding in progressive retinal atrophy and allied conditions (Par. 11:49), and, therefore, should never be used as an independent entity to establish a diagnosis of glaucoma.

9:25 The dilatation may be caused by a pressure paresis of the ciliary nerves, a paresis of the sphincter fibers because of edematous pressure, or an irritation of the sympathetic nerves. If tension is relieved early enough by medical or surgical intervention, the pupil may again become normally mobile and contracted. If the attack is prolonged and has produced synechiae (adhesions) at the root of the iris, or if atrophy of the iris has occurred, the pupil may remain dilated for life, even though the tension is normalized. The pupil dilatation is often one of the first signs noticed by the owner, as it produces a peculiar greenish blue hue (especially in cocker spaniels with acute congestive glaucoma). This color is thought to be an optical effect due to the turbidity of the optical media whereby the lens reflects light.

9:26 *Episcleral Vascularization* (Plate 9A). Episcleral vascularization, or congestion of the episcleral vessels, is a constant finding in tension increase. The vortex veins within the sclera are affected by the initial increase in tension. This makes it necessary for the anterior ciliary veins to take over their work, thus becoming distended in the process.

9:27 The conjunctival vessels also become injected and a mild degree of chemosis may accompany the change in the vessels. This engorgement is accentuated in the chronic and absolute stages by the inevitable globe enlargement (buphthalmos). When tension is restored to normal, the vessels tend to return to near normal size; the smaller ones disappear but seldom do any completely revert to their original caliber. The conjunctiva becomes "thinner" and even atrophic after a sustained tension increase.

9:28 *Loss of Vision.* Loss of vision, while due partly to failure of the owner to recognize the early stages, may also be due to failure on the part of the veterinary clinician to diagnose and treat the condition properly. If seen early, when there is little or only partial loss of vision, sight can often be preserved. When only one eye is glaucomatous, the dog may or may not show signs of blindness on the affected side. To test the ambulatory vision, a heavy black patch is placed over the normal eye (Par. 2:36) (Fig. 23). The dog is then observed as it moves through unfamiliar surroundings. When the tension increase if of long duration, and examination with the ophthalmoscope discloses extensive cupping and retinal atrophy, this test is not performed.

9:29 In the early acute congestive phase, the blindness that ensues is often of a transient nature, for when tension is normalized, vision is restored. The initial opacification of the ocular media contributes to the reduction in the vision, but ischemic changes in the retinal blood vessels, as a result of congestive changes in the retinal tissue, may also be a contributing factor. There may also be a pressure interference with transmission of impulses along the optic nerve fibers or a pressure interference with the function of the rods and cones.

9:30 In one instance, following normalization of tension, two weeks elapsed

before vision returned, although the ocular media was clear for most of that period. The return of vision was certainly dramatic, since all hope for sight had been abandoned. In other dogs, return of vision ensued within hours following tension relief, especially when this was accomplished by medical means. As a rule, the tension must be relieved within twenty-four to forty-eight hours following onset of acute congestive attacks and when tensions are 60 mm Hg or more, in order to prevent permanent damage and loss of vision.

9:31 *Buphthalmos (Hydrophthalmos).* The term hydrophthalmos or buphthalmos is applied to a glaucomatous eye when, under the influence of high tension, it has increased in size. These terms are used in human ophthalmology to denote infantile (congenital) glaucoma in which, because of the softness of the tissues, the gross distention of the eyeball is the main characteristic. While this is not found in the human adult, it is a constant clinical finding in canine glaucoma, whether it be primary or secondary, probably because the canine eye contains more elastic fibers. These terms are used synonymously; the French and English preferring "hydrophthalmos," with "buphthalmos" being more commonly used in this country.

9:32 Enlargement of the globe is a gradual although often rapid process. The full dilatation of the pupil, in the early stage of tension increase, gives to the eye an appearance of enlargement beyond that which is actually present. However, within a few weeks the globe may increase in size, with the cornea increasing in all dimensions and the eyeball appearing exophthalmic. As the buphthalmos increases, the eye develops an unpleasant appearance and is subjected to other inflammatory processes (Fig. 131).

9:33 *Cupping of the Optic Disc* (Fig. 132 A, B). Since the lamina cribosa, that portion of the sclera which is perforated by the optic nerve, is the most yielding area of the fibrous coat (Par. 6:172), it is pressed backward, producing a depression or cupping of the optic nerve head which is recognizable with the ophthalmoscope when the ocular media is clear. Ordinarily, this is not an early finding but it has been seen distinctly in dogs a few days following an acute attack. It is most readily seen in the blind, but clear, glaucomatous eye. For the normally myopic eye, a minus 3 lens of the ophthalmoscope is used first (Par. 2:50), with changes in diopters being made to view the fundus most clearly. In the case of subluxation of the lens, when attempting to visualize the fundus around the border of the lens, a plus 7 or 8 lens is used. In cupping, the blood vessels appear to drop over the edge of the optic disc and are only faintly seen at the bottom of the depression.

9:34 Recently a new study[9] proposes that the pathology of all "glaucomatous cupping" is mainly loss of tissue due to degeneration of nerve fiber and collagen and that there is a degenerative effect of vitreous on exposed collagen and nerve fiber. The vitreous degenerative effect on collagen and nerve fiber is proposed as the primary factor in "cupping" with increased intraocular pressure and vascular obstruction playing secondary or contributing roles.

9:35 *Atrophy of the Optic Disc and Retina.* More often than not, atrophy of the optic disc accompanies the cupping. The disc becomes grayish white

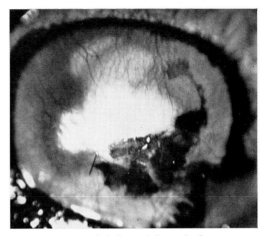

Fig. 131. Buphthalmic globe with glaucomatous pannus, pigment, and corneal dystrophy.

and few, if any, vessels can be seen emerging from it. The retina also becomes atrophic and nearly devoid of vessels.

9:36 *Iris Atrophy.* In the chronic and absolute types, glaucomatous changes are evident in the iris. It appears atrophic and thin, especially at the pupillary border (sphincter muscle area) (Plate 9D). In time, this area appears darker, patchy, and riddled with holes. Pigmentary deposits may be found on the anterior lens surface or free in the anterior chamber itself. In well-established cases with obscure histories, it is difficult to determine if extensive iris atrophy is the result, or the possible cause, of the tension increase (Par. 9:72).

Classification

A. Primary Glaucoma
B. Secondary Glaucoma
C. Congenital Glaucoma

9:37 Simply stated, and for all practical purposes, glaucoma may be classified as: (*a*) primary—in which the abnormal elevation of intraocular pressure occurs without other antecedent intraocular disease; (*b*) secondary—in which the abnormal elevation of intraocular pressure occurs as a complication of some other disease or damage to the eye; and (*c*) congenital—in which the abnormal elevation of intraocular pressure occurs as a result of some developmental malformation of the eye.

9:38   *Absolute* glaucoma, or blindness, is the end stage in any glaucoma. It need not be included in any classification, nor is it possible to do so in many instances in the dog for reasons previously mentioned (Par. 9:16).

General Considerations

9:39   A diagnosis of primary glaucoma is made when there are no discernible secondary conditions within the eye which could lead to an increase in tension. In other words, the cause of the tension increase cannot be definitely determined. In man, none of the many theories has adequately explained all cases of glaucoma. Two principal schools of thought or theories, the neurovascular and the mechanical, are proposed to explain the mechanism of primary glaucoma.

9:40   1) *The Neurovascular Theory.* This theory assumes that the disease results from an abnormality in the ocular circulation, which might occur on a local basis within the eye or as a consequence of a disturbance in the general circulatory system of the body as a whole. Contributing factors include disorders of the hypothalamic region, the autonomic nervous system, and the endocrine system.

9:41   2) *The Mechanical Theory.*

This theory assumes that an actual blockage to the drainage mechanism is the cause; it is based upon concepts established largely by gonioscopy. Many ophthalmologists are of the opinion that a combination of the two factors may cause the elevation in tension.

A. *Primary Glaucoma*[6]

9:42   *Breed Incidence.* Primary glaucoma is found almost exclusively in one breed of dogs, the cocker spaniel, indicating a hereditary predisposition. Lovekin[5] more recently bears this out by the discovery of manifest glaucoma in three generations of cocker spaniels of a single lineage, and in three other individuals of two separate lineages in which glaucoma was found in antecedents of the dogs examined. Several other breeds mentioned by Lovekin as possibly being afflicted with a primary type of glaucoma, *e.g.* wire fox terriers, may, in my opinion, have well been secondary types (subluxated lens) (Par. 9:55), in which the secondary cause was not discernible at the time the diagnosis was made.

9:43   In man glaucoma may be inherited as a dominant or recessive characteristic. In the study of several large series of persons with primary glaucoma that had one or more relatives affected with the disease, 13.7 to 17.8 per cent had a hereditary history.

9:44   *Sex Incidence.* In our series the ratio of females to males was 3:1. In Lovekin's series[5] the incidence of primary glaucoma was higher in males than in females, but the sample was relatively small. In man this form of glaucoma is reported to attack women more often than men.

9:45   *Eye Predilection.* There is a definite predilection for an initial left eye involvement in primary glaucoma. In one series the left eye was afflicted first in twice as many dogs as had an initial right eye involvement. This 2:1 ratio also resembles the ratio recorded in man.

9:46 *Age Incidence.* Primary glaucoma is a disease of middle and advancing age in both the cocker spaniel breed and in man. In our series the ages ranged from three and one-half to ten years. Lovekin[5] reports an age span of six to thirteen in this breed.

9:47 *Weather Incidence.* There is an obvious connection between weather conditions and the incidence of acute congestive attacks of glaucoma in man. Nearly twice as many attacks occur in northern cities during the cold months of October through March as in the warmer six-month period. When the dates of acute congestive attacks in cocker spaniels in our series could be determined, a near identical ratio was discovered. In Lovekin's study[5] all acute attacks occurred between October and May.

9:48 *Second Eye Involvement.* The time interval between the attack in the first eye and that in the second varies from a few days to two years. Nearly all second eye involvements will take place within one year. It has been well established that in man the second eye is especially susceptible to an acute attack of primary, shallow-chamber angle glaucoma following such an attack in the first eye.

9:49 *Mechanism and Theory of Cause.* In lieu of the overwhelming single breed incidence of primary acute congestive glaucoma in the dog, it is believed that a breed and familial predisposition is present. Anatomical factors may possibly contribute to this predisposition.

9:50 In man, there is strong evidence to support the theory that a narrow angle between the iris and the cornea predisposes to attacks of acute congestive glaucoma, the narrow angle thus offering an obstruction to the escape of the intraocular liquids. Acute congestive glaucoma is now being referred to as acute narrow-angle glaucoma in this country, but it is still not known if the angle is congenitally narrow or narrow as a result of some previous attacks.

9:51 Evidence obtained from gonioscopic studies[5, 7] in the cocker spaniel favors the definite possibility that a narrow iris angle predisposes to acute congestive attacks in certain individuals within the breed. A narrow or closed angle was found in both the affected and still unaffected eyes of those individual dogs in which this examination was possible.

B. *Secondary Glaucoma[7]*

9:52 A classification of secondary glaucoma is made when the abnormal elevation of intraocular pressure occurs as a complication of some other disease or damage to the eye. The mechanism of secondary glaucoma is fairly well understood, in that both neurovascular and mechanical factors enter into its production, either separately or together in the same eye.

9:53 Secondary glaucoma can affect any breed because of its multiplicity of causes. However, it is more apt to involve those breeds subjected to subluxation and luxation of the lens since this condition is the leading cause of a secondary tension rise in the dog. Secondary glaucoma occurs with far more frequency than does the primary form.

9:54   *Causes.* I have recognized eight causes for secondary glaucoma. It is not always possible to determine accurately the secondary cause for the increase in tension. In many instances it becomes evident from the history and time element that the disease has passed through the acute and chronic phases into the absolute (blind) stage without known secondary factors affecting the tension rise. Thus, the position and condition of the lens, intraocular adhesions, and iris pathology possibly present in the old glaucomatous eye may be the result of, rather than the cause of the glaucoma.

9:55   1) *Subluxation and Luxation of the Lens.* It is believed that luxation occurs when the ligamentous attachment of the lens is completely disrupted and when it has vacated the patellar fossa (Plate 9C and Fig. 146); subluxation occurs when the ligamentous breakdown is partial and displacement incomplete (Plate 9B and Figs. 143, 144 and 145).

9:56   In man, a number of mechanisms have been suggested as the cause of glaucoma secondary to partial or complete dislocation of the lens. The lens coming in contact with the ciliary processes may mechanically produce an irritative vasomotor reaction with edema, increased permeability, and increased aqueous formation. If the lens is subluxated forward, the angle of the anterior chamber may be partly blocked by the root of the iris pressing against the cornea. If the lens is completely luxated into the anterior chamber, it may block the pupillary space. Also, a dislocated lens may set up a uveitis which in turn leads to secondary glaucoma. Others believe that a pupillary block occurs when vitreous is pushed into the pupillary space by the posterior dislocation of the lens.

9:57   Secondary glaucoma resulting from subluxation of the lens is known to be familial. The genealogical tree of a family in which there were many cases of glaucoma associated with subluxation of the lens has been reported.

9:58   Although there are a few early accounts of luxation of the lens in animals, the first significant report, from the standpoint of selective breed incidence, showed it to be predominant in the pure bred wire-haired fox terrier and sealyham.[10]

9:59   In a classical work on subluxation and luxation of the lens in dogs, the condition was encountered in only the same two breeds, 90 per cent being in the wire-haired fox terrier and 10 per cent in sealyhams. However, these figures were not considered to be significant because they resembled the breed population ratios. In over 100 cases observed, no animal was under three years of age and the sexes were divided about equally (males, 56 per cent; females, 44 per cent). When first examined, 62 per cent of the animals were bilaterally affected and 38 per cent unilaterally.

9:60   The study[10] indicated that lenticular displacement is a primary affection and is hereditable, *i.e.*, certain organic defects are inherited which terminate specifically in a defective zonule; also, that displacement of the lens is probably often precipitated by trauma but, before displacement occurs, some degree of genetic instability must be present in the suspensory apparatus.

9:61   That the disease is hereditable is presumed[11] from the following circumstances: (1) the preponderance of bilateral cases (60 per cent); (2) the restricted and almost universal occurrence of the disease in the two named breeds of dogs; and (3) the indicated familial tendency. No figures are given as to the incidence of secondary glaucoma, but all cases, with one exception in which no trace of a lens could be found at necropsy, were associated with luxation of the lens into the anterior chamber.

9:62 Our series over the years includes an equally significant number of wire-haired terrier and sealyhams, but other breeds have been found to develop secondary glaucoma as the direct result of lens displacement. Included in this series are Welsh terriers, smooth-haired fox terriers, toy terriers, Manchester terriers, terriers of mixed breeding, Welsh corgis, chihuhuas, basset hounds and cocker spaniels. The range in all breeds afflicted varied from four to eight years of age.

9:63 In the cocker spaniel breed, it is not always possible to learn whether the glaucoma precipitates the lens luxation or vice versa. Certainly some of these cases will be primary in origin. Then, through long, continued tension increase, with resultant buphthalmos and stretching of the ocular structures, the lens suspensory apparatus is weakened, with a subluxation as the sequela. Primary cases of acute congestive glaucoma, which are untreated or fail to respond to treatment, can be observed to progress through stages of increased buphthalmos with eventual subluxation or luxation.

9:64 In other cases in the cocker spaniel which were seen early in the course of the disease, the lens displacement was known to have precipitated the tension rise. Trauma and a possible breed predisposition may be the responsible factors.

9:65 *Clinical Signs.* Since patients are presented during all stages of glaucoma, the clinical manifestations may include; (1) subluxation of the lens in any direction; (2) luxation into the anterior chamber; and (3) luxation into the vitreous humor. The degree of buphthalmos attending tension increase will, of course, depend upon the duration of the attack.

9:66 A corneal opacity often accompanies the lens displacement. Opacity was reported in all cases of luxation in one series.[10] In 87 per cent of another series,[11] corneal changes varied from a slight localized opacity to a diffuse vascularized keratitis. When an opacity is localized near the center of the cornea, the anterior pole of the lens can be observed to lie in contact with the endothelium of the cornea. The whole lens may be firmly adhered to the cornea in some instances. A striate keratitis has been observed in others with buphthalmos. It has been suggested[11] that most corneal lesions originate externally, affecting progressively the epithelium and subjacent corneal layers, and are caused by the affected animals blundering into obstacles because of the defective vision occurring after lens displacement.

9:67 The ease of diagnosing lens displacement, with or without secondary glaucoma, is again dependent upon the severity of the displacement. In the early stages, the only sign may be a distinct tremor of the iris, with movement of the head or eyes. This is known as iridodonesis (Par. 2:25) and results when the iris no longer has a smooth resting place on the anterior capsule of the lens. If the pupil is dilated, the periphery of the lens may be readily seen as a silver gray line and the zonules may often be seen still clinging to the lens capsule. Examination in a dark or semi-darkened room with magnification and focal illumination will materially aid in the diagnosis. Use of a Wood's light in a dark room will effect a green fluorescence of the lens which usually makes diagnosis simple. A displaced lens will become cataractous in time and, as transparency is lost, diagnosis is simplified (Figs. 143, 147).

9:68   It must be concluded that lens displacement is by far the most important cause of secondary glaucoma in the dog. The clinician should be highly suspicious that a subluxation is present if a middle aged dog of one of the aforementioned breeds is presented with a watery, sensitive eye. The acute congestive symptoms of glaucoma may not be present at the initial examination, and the tension increase may be transient, but—invariably, at some time during the course of lens displacement, a secondary glaucoma will be present.

9:69   2) *Uveitis.* Glaucoma secondary to intraocular inflammation (uveitis) is probably the next most common type of secondary glaucoma.

9:70   Posterior synechiae resulting from an iritis are most frequently the cause of tension increase. A complete adhesion of the pupillary margin of the iris to the anterior lens capsule (iris bombé) (Par. 7:37) (Fig. 123) will result in an absence of circulation of aqueous through the pupil, producing an increased pressure in the posterior chamber. The middle part of the iris will protrude forward, as the root and pupillary border are fixed. The lens diaphragm is also pushed forward. Due to the pressure of the iris root against the

cornea, the chamber angle becomes blocked (Fig. 132C). Thus, what aqueous that does manage to reach the anterior chamber no longer has an exit.

9:71   Atrophy of the iris as a sequela to uveitis (Par. 7:38) can lead to a secondary glaucoma (Plate 7E). The sloughing pigment and iris debris clogs the drainage angle thus slowing down the aqueous drainage through the trabeculum.

9:72   3) *Essential Iris Atrophy.* I have seen several cases in which it was believed that the iris atrophy was primary to the glaucoma. An essential progressive iris atrophy is described in man in which iris tissue is lost in all layers. This tissue loss results in a loss of the resorption capacity of the iris and tends to block the angle with iris debris in the manner described (Par. 9:71).

9:73   It is necessary to see iris atrophy in the early stage in the dog in order to brand the atrophy as the cause of the glaucoma. As pointed out earlier (Par. 9:36), tension increase of some duration will produce iris atrophy. A diagnosis of essential iris atrophy will always prove difficult in the dog, but the clinician's suspicions might be aroused if an extensive iris atrophy without full pupil dilatation or without iris-lens adhesions is seen, and yet tension is increased.

9:74   4) *Injury and Infection.* Adhesions as a sequela to trauma or endophthalmitis will, of course, block the drainage mechanism, with secondary glaucoma as the result. The trauma or infection may precede the tension increase by some weeks. As a rule, this type of glaucoma is the most refractory to medical or surgical treatment.

9:75   5) *Postsurgical (cataract ex-*

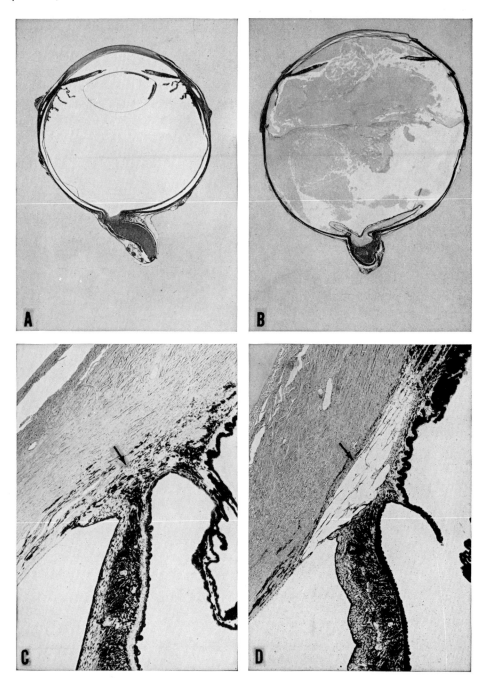

Fig. 132.   Canine glaucoma. *A. Section* (× 2) of the left eye of a dog with moderately severe glaucoma. Note spherical outline of the eye, occlusion of the filtration angle and cupping of the optic disc. *B.* Absolute glaucoma in the right eye of the same dog as A (× 2). Buphthalmos, severe cupping of the optic disc, disorganization of contents of globe. *C.* Filtration angle (× 35) of same eye as A. Note occlusion (arrow) AFIP 717599. Contributor: Dr. Leon Z. Saunders. *D.* Normal filtration angle, eye of a dog (× 35). Compare with C. (Smith and Jones, *Veterinary Pathology.* Courtesy: Lea and Febiger.)

traction). Secondary glaucoma following operations for cataracts is not uncommon. It was reported in 0.64 to 3.0 per cent of human patients after extracapsular extraction or discission. The percentage is less following intracapsular extraction.

9:76   There are several principal reasons for secondary glaucoma following operations for cataracts. The most important factor is delayed reformation of the anterior chamber which, in turn, is due to fistulization. Iris prolapse, incarceration of lens capsule, long standing or repeated hyphema, or the presence of many cortical lens remnants will cause fistulization. Vitreous prolapse, with blockage of the angle or production of an iris bombé, is believed to be a cause of glaucoma. Postoperative iridocyclitis, epithelial ingrowth, and postoperative edema are additional causes.

9:77   Our series includes several cases which had been subjected to a lens discission procedure six months or more before, and several others that had an extracapsular extraction performed. One of these was afflicted one month following a surgical procedure. At that time it had vitreous in its shallow anterior chamber. Another had been operated on three years before, but considerable lens debris remained in the anterior chamber.

9:78   6) *Lenticular Intumescence.* Secondary glaucoma due to lens swelling (intumescence) occurs in eyes predisposed to acute attack by virtue of a narrow drainage angle (Par. 9:51). By means of gonioscopy, it was found that the angle of the eye opposite the one with lenticular swelling was of the narrow type.

9:79   In swelling of the lens, during development of a cataract, there is a disposition to glaucoma due to the shallowing of the anterior chamber with a decrease in the circumlental space which permits other factors to block the angle. The swelling may even press the iris against the trabecular wall.

9:80   Young cocker spaniels with a history of rapid development of juvenile cataract are the most likely candidates for this type of secondary glaucoma. Those cases seen have exhibited changes that included a "steamy" cornea, immobile iris, shallow anterior chamber, swollen cataractous lens, episcleral vessel congestion, and tension well above normal.

9:81   7) *Hypermature Cataract and*

Plate 9.

A. Acute congestive glaucoma. Note congestion and ejection of the conjunctival and episcleral vessels and dilatation of the pupil.

B. Subluxated lens and secondary glaucoma. Lens is displaced to the superior position with the lower border visible as an aphakic crescent.

C. Luxation of the lens into the anterior chamber. Note bluish "cast" to lens.

D. Absolute glaucoma with secondary iris atrophy.

E. Absolute glaucoma with secondary intraocular hemorrhage. Note congestion and ejection of the conjunctival and episcleral vessels, dilatation of the pupil (above the blood level), and bluish "cast" to the sclera (denotes thinning).

F. Iridencleisis bleb two weeks post operatively. Small blood clot on the anterior capsule of the lens is absorbing.

G. Basal, peripheral iridectomy opposite 10:00 o'clock.

H. Iridectomy (base of pupillary margin). Post operative appearance following correction of secondary glaucoma resulting from an iris bombé.

Plate 9

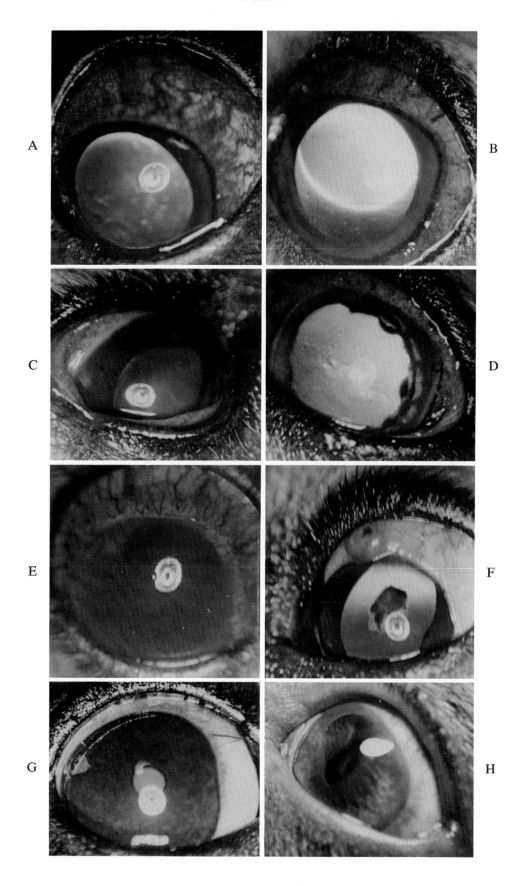

Spontaneous Lens Capsule Rupture. After passing through the intumescent or immature state, cataract progresses through the mature into the hypermature. In this stage, the cortex may become liquified, as may the entire nucleus in a younger individual. All that remains is a sac filled with milky fluid (Morgagnian cataract) (Plate 10D) due to the action of a lytic ferment. Only a thin transparent capsule is left, which will often rupture spontaneously. Three possible causes of glaucoma following spontaneous lens-capsule rupture have been listed: (1) chemical irritation by lens substance; (2) increased protein content of the aqueous which tends to lessen the osmotic differential between the aqueous and the blood serum; and (3) obstruction of the trabecular spaces by particles of lens substance. The first is the only condition which appears to be present in every case.

9:82　　The incidence of hypermature cataract formation is in proportion to the increased incidence of juvenile cataract development in numerous breeds (Par. 10:25). The presence of glaucomatous changes associated with a history of long-standing cataract and loss of vision is suggestive of hypermaturity. Upon examination of the lens, the nucleus will be seen lying in the lower part and, due to the liquification of the cortex, a fundic reflection will be discernible (Plate 10D). Ophthalmoscopy, utilizing the plus 8–12 lens, will bring fundus detail into view.

9:83　　When a hypermature cataract is surgically removed (intracapsular extraction), it resembles a deflated football bladder.

9:84　　8) *Intraocular Neoplasm.* Secondary glaucoma resulting from drainage angle occlusion by a uveal tract tumor may be expected in those eyes in which the growth is allowed to progress (Par. 7:76).

Medical and Surgical Treatment[12]

9:85　　The treatment of glaucoma, whether it be primary or secondary, is both medical and surgical. In the dog, however, medical treatment as the sole means of controlling tension has proved unsatisfactory. It is not because medical treatment fails in every instance to control tension but because, even though drugs may be effective, pet owners become lax in treatment and fail to recognize the return of tension increases. Miotics and a carbonic anhydrase inhibitor drug often must be used continuously, one or more times a day, in order to maintain a normal tension, and failure to do so results in further loss of vision and eventual blindness. Also, most owners are reluctant to assume the responsibility of daily care and observation necessary over a period of years. It has been our experience that, in most instances where control depended upon drugs, eventually those drugs failed and surgery was necessary. Usually, vision had been progressively lost by that time.

9:86　　We now prefer a surgical procedure in nearly all cases of glaucoma, but use medical treatment to normalize the tension whenever possible, both as an emergency measure in acute congestive attacks and to facilitate the surgical procedures. Medical treatment is also needed, in some instances, to augment surgical procedures.

Medical Treatment

9:87　　The non-operative treatment for primary glaucoma consists primarily of the use of <u>miotics</u> (Par. 3:32). If effective in constricting the pupil, miotics reduce intraocular tension by (1) opening up the cornea-iris angle, (2) opening the posterior venous channels, (3) constricting the blood supply into the ciliary body, and (4) allowing more surface area of the iris to absorb the aqueous humor.

9:88   The action of miotics for relief of glaucoma is largely dependent upon the type of glaucoma and the mobility of the iris. For example, if a complete posterior synechia (iris bombé) is present, there would be little effect as regards the opening of the drainage angle.

9:89   The two miotics most commonly used in the past, eserine and pilocarpine (Par. 3:33), never satisfactorily controlled acute congestive attacks in the dog. However, with the advent of di-isopropyl fluorophosphate (DEP) and, more recently, demacarium bromide (<u>Humorsol</u>) (Par. 3:34), medical control of certain types of glaucoma is possible. Combined with the use of a carbonic anhydrase inhibitor (Par. 3:66) tensions of 60 to 80 mm Hg may be lowered to normal within twelve to twenty-four hours.

9:90   Carbonic anhydrase inhibitors act on the eye by inhibiting the formation of aqueous humor. They have no effect on the outflow and so should be used in combination with miotics. They are synergistic with miotics since they act on the two different mechanisms producing intraocular pressure, secretion of aqueous fluid, and decreased outflow. By lowering the intraocular tension through decreased secretion, miosis is achieved more readily by miotics; thus the angle is unblocked and drainage can occur.

9:91   While carbonic anhydrase inhibitors have been effective for months into the years in some cases, in others the effect has been maintained for only a week or two. These preparations are important as a preoperative medication in all types of glaucoma since their use makes possible an operation on a softer, less inflamed eye with less likelihood of complications.

9:92   The dosage of carbonic anhydrase inhibitors varies with the preparation used. Familiarity with one product is recommended because of possible side effects (nausea, vomiting, drowsiness, increased urination). Cardrase* is used as follows: average 20 to 30 pound dog 62.5 mg every eight hours for three doses, followed by the same dose (or less) at twelve-hour intervals. The dose will vary with individuals and is also dependent upon the type and severity of the glaucoma.

9:93   Floropryl 0.1 per cent (DFP)** instillations are made hourly (4 to 6 times) and then once or twice a day thereafter to maintain miosis. This preparation is in an oil base, is hydroscopic, and is rendered ineffective if moisture enters the bottle.

9:94   Humorsol 0.25 per cent*** has an aqueous base, is more stable, and exerts an even more powerful miotic effect in the dog. Fewer instillations are required and once miosis is achieved it may be maintained with as little as one instillation per day or every other day.

9:95   The importance of this combination therapy (a miotic and a carbonic anhydrase inhibitor) in normalizing tension, thus preventing further visual loss and preparing a softer eye for surgery, cannot be overestimated. If surgery is rejected or the animal is very old, the combination may be used

---

* Upjohn Co., Kalamazoo, Mich.
** Merck Sharp & Dohme, Philadelphia, Pa.
*** Merck Sharp & Dohme, Philadelphia, Pa.

as long as it proves effective or is without undesirable side effects.

9:96 Of late the intravenous use of mannitol 20 per cent (2 gm/kg) has been used to help lower tension prior to surgery when carbonic anhydrase inhibitors have failed to do so. Intravenous urea* 30 per cent (1.0 to 1.5 gm/kg) and oral glycerine (1.5 cc/kg) are also effective in lowering tension temporarily.

9:97 The retrobulbar injection of pure grain alcohol (2 cc) may be tried for relief of pain and a possible reduction in tension in absolute (blind) glaucoma. When surgical procedures are rejected or fail, or for the practitioner who anticipates enucleation of a blind, glaucomatous eye, there is nothing to lose by attempting this procedure. It may be repeated at intervals, if necessary, and is easily performed.

9:98 Under short-duration barbiturate anesthesia, a 1¼ to 1½ inch, 22-gauge needle is inserted to a point just behind the posterior surface of the globe (Fig. 133). Several approaches may be selected but I prefer to insert the needle through the conjunctiva, medial and ventral to the globe along the inferior orbital ridge following, by feel, the cartilaginous orbit. The globe should be fixed in the opposite quadrant with fixation forceps. After injection, the needle is withdrawn and a slight rotary pressure is exerted on the globe through the closed lids in order to promote thorough diffusion within the cone.

Surgical Treatment

9:99 As pointed out previously, the treatment of choice for glaucoma, regardless of type, is practically always

* Urevert. Travenol Labs, Inc., Morton Grove, Ill.

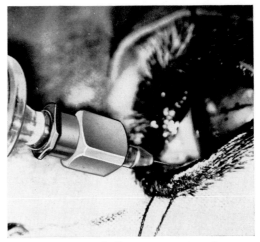

Fig. 133. Retrobulbar injection. Needle is inserted along side the medial-ventral aspect of the globe.

surgical. There is, however, no one surgical procedure to care for all glaucomas. A careful examination and an accurate classification is necessary in order to determine the type of procedure that is best suited for each case.

9:100 The prime objective in the surgical treatment of glaucoma is to secure a lower tension and preserve vision; and second, if the condition be absolute, to preserve the integrity of the globe—in other words, to avoid enucleation. Since so many glaucomas in the dog are in the absolute stage before the dog is presented, pet owners are usually pleased if, through surgery, the dog's eye is rendered painless and the buphthalmos is checked. They much prefer this to enucleation and closing of the orbit, which is almost inevitable if the buphthalmos is allowed to progress. For these reasons, surgery of the blind eye is practical in the dog.

9:101 It has been said that enucleation of a glaucomatous eye in the dog will prevent glaucoma in the second eye. This has not been our experience (Par. 9:48). In the past, attacks of glaucoma in the second eye, following enucleation of the first, occurred in several instances within a matter of days and often within months.

9:102   This section on surgical treatment is written only for the purpose of enumerating the procedures that have been employed in the dog and briefly describing the techniques as they apply to the various types of glaucoma. The *General Considerations for Eye Surgery* (Chapter 3) should be taken into account before the clinician makes the decision to engage in this specialized facet of canine ophthalmology.

9:103   The operations performed in the dog may be classified as follows: iridectomy (peripheral, basal, prophylactic); filtering cicatrix (iridencleisis, sclero-iridencleisis, Elliot trephine); tube implant filtration; cyclodialysis; cyclodiathermy; and lens ablation (intracapsular, extracapsular).

Iridectomy

9:104   This operation is indicated within the first few days of an attack of primary glaucoma. If postponed, it is apt to fail because peripheral anterior synechiae will have begun to develop. In primary glaucoma with a narrow or closed drainage angle the performance of a basal (iris root) iridectomy will re-establish circulation to the trabeculum (Plate 9G).

9:105   An iridectomy is also the procedure of choice in the re-establishment of circulation from the posterior to the anterior chamber in an iris bombé (Plate 9H). A peripheral excision through the center and/or pupillary border of the iris will suffice, provided the drainage angle is still patent. An iridectomy from pupillary border through the base will be indicated more often.

9:106   A prophylactic basal iridectomy (Plate 9G) may be performed on the normal eye in those cases of primary, closed angle glaucoma in which it is felt that the second eye will become involved in time. In our experience this has prevented an attack in the second eye in several instances but has had no effect in the prevention in several others. These failures, however, may have been due to a poorly executed procedure. In any event, the decision to perform a prophylactic surgical procedure on a normal eye is a serious one.

Filtering Cicatrix

9:107   Filtering cicatrix operations have as their object the formation of a permanent filtering cicatrix at or near the sclerocorneal junction through which the excess of aqueous fluid filters out under the conjunctiva (Plate 9F). While this has been generally assumed to be the mechanism whereby tension is reduced, considerable evidence to the contrary has been produced.

9:108   It has been concluded that the persistence of a small area of conjunctival edema after iridencleisis does not definitely demonstrate that the scar is the site of a real filtration. Scars are often flat and seem to exclude the possibility of any filtration, and yet the tension reduction is excellent. Iridencleisis may lower and normalize the ocular tension by inducing complex neurovascular modifications at the level of the anterior uvea.

9:109   In the majority of cases in one series (man) of successful iridencleisis operations, the resistance to aqueous fluid outflow was brought down to normal range and the operative area did not show any signs of fluid filtration into subconjunctival tissue spaces. These findings suggest that the action of the iridencleisis consists in enhancing or re-establishing the function of the normal outflow channels. Only in about one-fourth of those cases did a permanent bleb form.

9:110 Following iridencleisis, we have seen functional blebs remain a long time, but the scars usually became flat eventually. In those with flattened scars, the tension remained normal in some but became elevated again in others. However, in all in which the bleb appeared functional, the tension remained normal.

9:111 The indications for filtering cicatrix procedures include: primary, closed angle glaucoma; secondary glaucoma caused by a iris bombé in which peripheral anterior synechiae have obliterated the drainage angle; and, secondary glaucoma due to injury and adhesions in which the angle is closed.

9:112 When the iris becomes atrophic or degenerated, an iridencleisis is more likely than not to fail. Also, an iridencleisis is not liable to be successful in those cases in which a displacement of the lens is the cause of the secondary glaucoma.

9:113 *The Operation.* Many variations of iridencleisis or iris inclusion operations are described. Our technique has been varied to include: (1) incarceration of one tag of iris following a split of the iris from base to sphincter; (2) incarceration of both tags following the split; (3) excision of a wedge of iris before incarceration of a tag; (4) suturing the tag to the episcleral tissue; (5) incarceration of a tag through a trephine hole (sclerectomy); (6) incarceration, through the wound and into the anterior chamber, of a limbal based

half thickness scleral flap, in addition to the iris tag inclusion; and (7) application of Gelfilm* to the incarcerated tag and incision site.

9:114 The principal steps in the iridencleisis operation are:
1) The conjunctival flap is prepared, starting about 8 mm from the limbus, undermining the conjunctiva so that the sclera is bared. The undermining should extend to the limbus in the central portion of the flap only.
2) The incision, 4 to 5 mm, through the sclera into the anterior chamber is made about 1 mm behind the limbus. Patency may be enhanced by making the incision with an electrocautery or subjecting the wound edges to heat cautery.
3) The iris is allowed to prolapse or is grasped with iris forceps or a dull iris hook and brought to the outside. Holding the iris with forceps on each side, an incision is made from the base through the sphincter muscle and free border and one or both tags are pulled to the edge of the scleral incision where it is incarcerated. If only one tag is used, the second is allowed to return to its position in the anterior chamber.
4) The conjunctival flap is replaced over the incarcerated tag and sutured in place with 5–0 chromic catgut. A drop of atropine solution (2 per cent) is instilled and the eye bandaged.

9:115 In order to secure permanent filtration from the anterior chamber to the immediate subconjunctival spaces, a sterile, nonantigenic, absorbable film made from pig gelatin has been utilized (Gelfilm*). When dry, it looks and feels like cellophane, but when wet it assumes a soft rubbery consistency which molds well to any body surface. Its absorption requires from one to three months, and an opening or "en-

* Gelfilm, Upjohn Co., Kalamazoo, Mich.

velope" remains between the conjunctiva and sclera.

9:116   Trephination, without incarceration of the iris, may be considered when the iris becomes atrophic or degenerated. There is a difference of opinion as to whether the results produced by trephining are due to fistulization or other factors.

9:117   Briefly, in trephining, a conjunctival flap is first prepared, extending the dissection to include the corneal epithelium for several millimeters in the center of the flap. A 2 to 3 mm trephine is then used to remove a disc which includes one-half cornea and one-half sclera. An iridectomy or iridotomy should be combined with the trephination. The conjunctival flap is replaced and sutured in the manner described for iridencleisis.

Tube Implant Filtration (Fig. 134)

9:118   A method, still in the investigational stage, is the use of an inert

material (silicone) to establish permanent filtration. A piece of Silastic tubing has been placed between the anterior chamber and subconjunctival region in several dozen cases. The Silastic tube* is anchored to the episcleral tissue with 6–0 mersilene or catgut which has been preplaced through the end of the tube. Gelfilm is then placed on top of the tube and under the conjunctiva in the manner described (Par. 9:115), and the conjunctiva is replaced in the usual manner.

9:119   The use of an innocuous material which does not absorb should, theoretically, result in permanent patency. Generally, a good result was obtained on a short term follow-up of the series, but latent extrusion of the tube and tissue closure on the scleral side resulted in enough failures to warrant further study. Careful selection of cases, perfecting of the tube placement, and a

* Medical Silastic 373,   0.025″ × 0.050,″ Dow Corning, Midland, Mich.

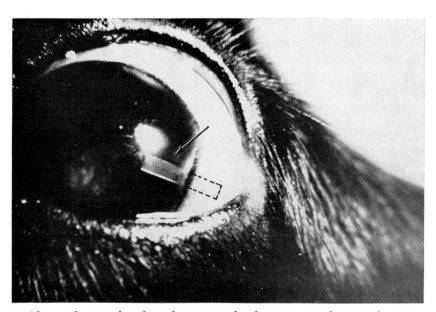

Fig. 134.   Silastic tube extending from the anterior chamber to an area between the conjunctiva and sclera. Dotted line denotes position of the tube on the scleral side.

long term follow up will be necessary before a true evaluation of this procedure can be made.

Cyclodialysis

9:120 This operation creates an artificial communication between the anterior chamber and the suprachoroidal space, thus forming a new channel for the escape of aqueous.

9:121 A cyclodialysis spatula is introduced through an incision in the bared sclera 5 to 7 mm from and parallel to the limbus. The blade is kept close to the sclera and advanced in a sweeping motion until its point appears in the anterior chamber. The root of the iris and ciliary body and thus detached, creating the channel. Überreiter[13] believes that this procedure is best suited to the dog, but he does not suggest the type of glaucoma in which it is indicated or most effective.

9:122 We have utilized cyclodialysis to compliment other procedures and when peripheral anterior synechiae are evident or suspected. The spatula may be introduced from the anterior chamber side to separate the iris root and ciliary body. In our experience, the operation by itself often fails to afford permanent reduction in tension. Considerable hemorrhage can be expected in association with this procedure.

Cyclodiathermy

9:123 By definition, cyclodiathermy is application of diathermic current to the ciliary body through the sclera by means of penetrating or nonpenetrating electrodes.

9:124 The exact mechanism of action of cyclodiathermy in lowering intraocular pressure is not completely understood. Whether it acts primarily to destroy the secretory function of the ciliary body by interfering with its vascular supply, or whether it serves to stimulate the formation of a new anastomotic group of vessels and thus effect overflow of aqueous fluid has not been established. Some (in man) advocate its use primarily when all other procedures have failed, while others are of the opinion that the procedure should be reserved for cases in which filtering operations are contraindicated, or in which outflow following a filtering procedure is mildly inadequate.

9:125 We have used cyclodiathermy successfully after one or more procedures have already been tried and failed to normalize tension. In other cases the procedure either failed to reduce tension, reduced it partially, or produced a hypotony which led to a phthisis bulbi (atrophy of the eyeball).

9:126 *The Operation.* While varying techniques for applying the electrodes have been described, we employed the same one in all eyes. A Miller electrosurgical unit (Fig. 28A) was used. The technique follows: (1) The eye is draped and fixed below with fixation forceps so that the upper portion of the globe is well exposed and the bulbar conjunctiva taut. (2) A 1.5 mm electrode is applied through the conjunctiva and into the sclera, 5 to 6 mm behind the upper limbus, and at 8 to 10 points evenly spaced to cover the upper half of the globe (Fig. 135). A millimeter rule may be used for the measurement. (3) With the electrode set at 1 (to produce coagulation), it is held in place for ten seconds at each application. (4) Atropine solution (2 per cent) and an antibiotic are instilled and the eye is bandaged for two days.

9:127 Occasionally, there will be a

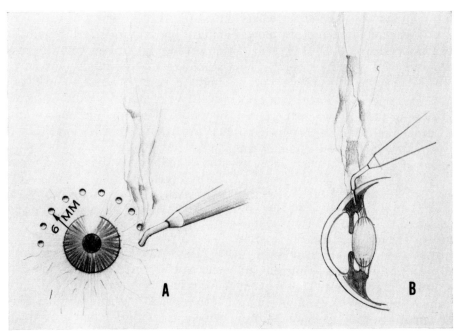

Fig. 135. Cyclodiathermy. A. Application of the electrode to the upper hemisphere of the globe. B. Side view showing position of the electrode in its relation to the ciliary body.

loss of fluid from some of the punctures, which is desirable. A moderate chemosis (edema of the conjunctiva) will be in evidence for several days following the procedure. This is alleviated by use of steroid drops or ointment. A secondary rise in tension may follow the operation but this soon subsides.

9:128   Cyclodiathermy is indicated for relief of tension in blind eyes only (absolute glaucoma). It is easily performed and may be repeated as needed. Buphthalmia often subsides after several weeks, and some eyes even return to normal size.

Lens Ablation

9:129   Lens extraction is recommended in glaucoma: (1) due to subluxation or luxation of the lens; (2) due to swelling or intumescence of the lens; (3) when it is secondary to lens-induced uveitis, *e.g.*, capsule rupture in hypermature cataracts; (4) when it is malignant, and (5) when due to acute iris block of an advanced nature when accompanied by a very shallow anterior chamber and a high tension which does not respond to medication. Malignant glaucoma is defined as one in which surgical intervention is promptly followed by a flat anterior chamber and an elevated tension, both of which are unresponsive to further measures.

9:130   The most frequent operation to be performed in canine glaucoma is removal of the lens, the displacement of which is responsible for the secondary tension rise. Intracapsular extraction is attempted in all instances of lens displacement. Occasionally, an extracapsular extraction results when, inadvertently, the capsule ruptures during extraction. This usually occurs when the lens is bound by adhesions.

9:131   Since lens displacement is directly responsible for a secondary tension rise, the surgery for the removal of the lens is specific for this type of secondary glaucoma. If performed properly, with meticulous attention to detail, the results achieved are generally excellent as regards affording permanent relief of tension. The most consistent results and the highest percentage of success following surgery are encountered in this type of glaucoma. It is important, however, that surgery be performed before the eye becomes too buphthalmic.

9:132 Useful vision may also be retained provided the lens ablation is performed before tension induced degenerative changes occur. As Knight[14] indicates, "it cannot be emphasized too strongly that if the dog with a dislocated lens is to retain useful aphakic vision, the extraction of the lens is best regarded as an operation of necessity as soon as the condition can be diagnosed; and for this reason diagnosis at the earliest stage is most important."

The Operation

9:133 (1) *Canthotomy* (Par. 4:11) (Fig. 40). The necessity for performing a canthotomy depends upon the amount of buphthalmos and the size of the palpebral fissure. If the eye is well exposed, a canthotomy is unnecessary.

9:134 (2) *Retrobulbar injection* (Par. 9:98) (Fig. 133). If additional anesthesia or further reduction of tension is desired, 2 cc of a 2 per cent procaine solution is injected into the region of the muscle cone. With the preoperative use of carbonic anhydrase inhibitors to lower tension and adequate general anesthesia, this step is no longer important.

9:135 (3) *Conjunctival flap* (limbal based). Approximately 5 mm from the upper limbus, the conjunctiva and Tenon's capsule is incised around the upper half of the eye to the sclera, and is dissected down to the limbus with knife and scissors.

9:136 (4) *Preliminary groove.* A half thickness incision or groove is made along the line of the contemplated section about 0.5 to 1.0 mm posterior to the limbus and near the base of the conjunctival flap. A No. 64 Beaver blade may be used, but, to eliminate all hemorrhage, an offset electroscalpel blade (Fig. 136) and the electrocautery (Par. 3:73) is preferred.

9:137 (5) *Preplaced sutures.* Five or six sutures (Par. 3:105) are preplaced at equal distance in the groove before the incision is made, thus eliminating the hazard of manipulating the collapsed open eye. The preplacement of sutures is extremely important in this operation. When entering the anterior chamber, there is usually an immediate presentation of vitreous because the hyaloid membrane (Par. 11:2) is ruptured at the time the lens displacement occurred. The post placing of sutures following lens extraction is not only difficult, but the excessive manipulation required will result in considerable loss of vitreous.

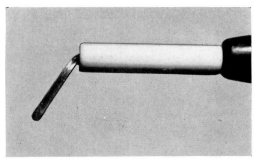

Fig. 136. Offset electroscalpel blade used to prepare scleral grooves.

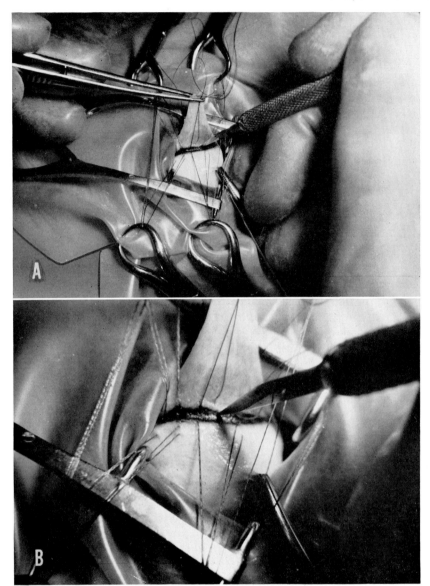

Fig. 137. Entry into the anterior chamber for lens ablation. *A.* Surgeon's view of the dorsal aspect of
the globe. Preplaced sutures are separated and held away from the scleral groove by towel forceps. Conjunctival flap is extended perpendicularly. Eyeball is fixed with rat tooth mosquito forceps attached to
the episclera. Knife incision is made through the center of the sclera groove into the angle of the anterior
chamber. *B.* Close up view.

9:138   The sutures (McLean type)
do not penetrate into the chambers of
the eye. The needle, starting at the base
of the anterior (epithelial) surface of the
conjunctival flap, passes through it. It
is then reversed and brought anteriorly
by catching the posterior scleral lip of
the groove, passing in the scleral tissue
to cross the groove just dorsal to its
depth. The anterior scleral lip of the
groove is then penetrated and the needle emerges at the limbus just opposite

the other end of the suture (inverted mattress suture). Each double strand of suture, where it is exposed in the groove, is picked up with an iris hook to form a loop. Each loop is separated and held away from the incision site by towel forceps or a suitable substitute (Fig. 137A).

9:139 (6) *Section.* With the eyeball fixed, a No. 65 Beaver blade is used to enter the angle of the anterior chamber on the scleral side (Fig. 137B). The incision is then extended with corneal scissors with care being taken not to cut the preplaced sutures. The section must be as adequate as is necessary to remove the entire lens without undue pressure. To minimize loss of vitreous there should be no pressure on the eye; thus, the speculum tension is reduced prior to enlarging the incision. This is best accomplished by having the assistant hold and elevate the end of the speculum, thus raising the blades and lids away from the globe.

9:140 (7) *Iridectomy.* A peripheral,

pupillary iridectomy may be performed to afford more working room for the extraction but this is rarely necessary. Rather, an intact iris is important to the "holding back" of the vitreous following extraction. If an iridectomy or iridotomy is performed, the use of the electrocautery for this purpose will prevent the hemorrhage that accompanies the scissor method.

9:141 (8) *Extraction.* A wire lens snare is used to encompass the posterior part of the lens, thus lifting the lens forward and dorsal to and partially through the incision site (Fig. 138). The lens is then steadied and held with smooth capsule forceps, while corneal scissors are used to cut clinging vitreous from the posterior capsule. Any vitreous is cleared from the incision site and is gently smoothed into the pupillary area.

9:142 (9) *Closure.* The preplaced sutures are drawn up and tied and an air bubble is injected into the anterior chamber with a hypodermic syringe or irrigating bulb and lacrimal needle. If

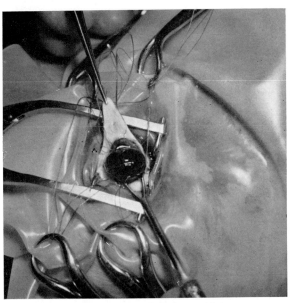

Fig. 138. Extraction of the lens with lens snare.

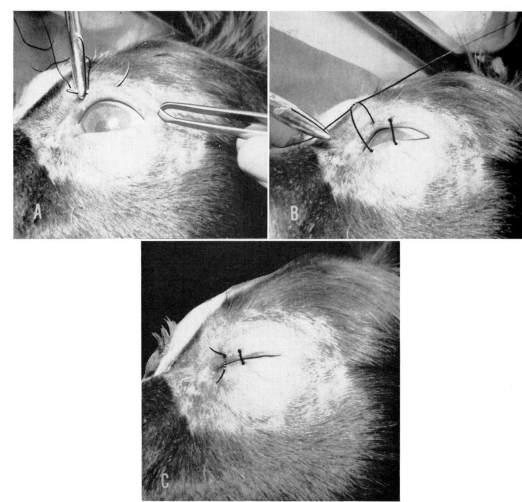

Fig. 139.   Mode of lid closure. A. Needle penetrates skin only.
   B. Mattress suture is continued to the lower lid prior to the tie. C. Completed lid closure. There is no suture contact with the cornea.

the closure is secure, the air bubble will serve to "blow back" the vitreous into its rightful chamber. Tenon's capsule and the conjunctiva are replaced and sutured with 5–0 chromic catgut. A drop of pilocarpine solution (2 per cent) and an antibiotic is instilled, a single mattress suture is placed to close the lids (Fig. 139), and a bandage is applied (Par. 3:81) (Fig. 31).

Postoperative Care (all glaucoma cases)
9:143   Proper postoperative care is exceedingly important following all intraocular procedures of the eye in the dog. Bandaging is important for the reasons elicited (Par. 3:80). Dressings may be changed daily or on alternate days with instillation of the antibiotic used following surgery. Bandaging may be discontinued after four or five days. The lid suture is removed a week following surgery and a steroid-antibiotic preparation may then be used several times a day to prevent neovascularization and to keep the eye "quiet."

9:144   The corneoscleral sutures are removed on the twelfth postoperative day. This is most easily accomplished by using eye tissue forceps and the tip of a No. 65 Beaver blade following good topical anesthesia. Only occasionally is tranquilization and/or general anesthesia necessary for suture removal. The conjunctival suture is left to absorb. Careful handling of the patient, freedom of excitement, and the use of protective collars (Fig. 140) for at least the first week are important during hospitalization.

9:145   The hospitalization period will vary from seven to fourteen days depending upon the type of surgery performed. Upon discharge the owner is instructed to continue the steroid-antibiotic preparation for about another week.

Postoperative Complications

9:146   Postoperative complications are most apt to occur as a result of faulty technique, or the selection of an improper procedure for the type and stage of glaucoma presented. However, even when the technique is apparently faultless and proper operation is selected, a certain percentage of operations are doomed to failure.

9:147   One author[15] reports a minimum of 15 per cent failure at the first operation, and at least 50 per cent at reoperation. He cautions against repeating a procedure which has failed once.

9:148   Glaucoma frequently leads to the formation of lens opacities which cannot be avoided. Lens opacities and cataract, however, may be hastened by operative trauma, and care must be exercised to avoid touching the lens during filtering procedures.

9:149   Other postoperative complications include: vitreous prolapse, wound separation, uveitis, late infection, filtration failures due to adhesions and fibrotic changes, lens displacement, retinal detachment, and phthisis bulbi —to name a few. Clotted blood remaining in the anterior chamber may cause major complications and failure. The use of the electrocautery for groove preparation and iridectomies, and controlling all hemorrhage attending a step before proceeding to the next, minimizes this possibility.

9:150   In summary, the surgical treatment of glaucoma in the dog is feasible provided the glaucoma is classified accurately, the proper operation is selected, and the technique is perfected. Permanent tension reduction to normal or below normal can be expected in more than half of all those operated, and a very high percentage of success can be expected in certain types, *e.g.*, lens displacement.

9:151   In general one or a combination of these procedures may be applicable to these glaucoma types.

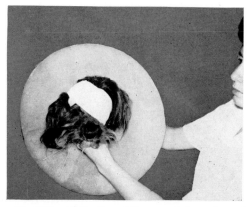

Fig. 140.   Protection of the operated eye through use of bandaging and a plastic collar.

TYPE	THERAPY
Primary Glaucoma	
Acute congestive (narrow angle)	Miotic; Carbonic anhydrase inhibitor Iridectomy (basal)
Chronic congestive (narrow angle)	Miotic; carbonic anhydrase inhibitor Filtering cicatrix
Secondary Glaucoma	
1. Subluxation and luxation	Miotic; carbonic anhydrase inhibitor Lens ablation
2. Uveitis (adhesions)	Carbonic anhydrase inhibitor Iridectomy Cyclodialysis Filtering cicatrix
3. Essential iris atrophy	Miotic; carbonic anhydrase inhibitor Trephination Tube implant
4. Injury and infection (adhesions)	Carbonic anhydrase inhibitor Iridectomy Cyclodialysis Filtering cicatrix
5. Postsurgical (cataract)	Carbonic anhydrase inhibitor Iridectomy; break adhesions; removal of lens debris
6. Lenticular Intumescence	Miotic; carbonic anhydrase inhibitor Lens ablation
7. Hypermature Cataract	Miotic; carbonic anhydrase inhibitor Lens ablation (intracapsular)
8. Intraocular Neoplasm	Enucleation
Absolute (blind) *Glaucoma*	As listed or; cyclodiathermy Retrobulbar alcohol

References

1. Troncoso, M. U.: *Gonioscopy*, Philadelphia, F. A. Davis Co., 1948.
2. Leber, T.: Cited by Troncoso, M. U.: *Gonioscopy*, Philadelphia, F. A. Davis Co., p. 57, 1948.
3. Friendenwald, J. S. and Pierce, H. T.: Circulation of the Aqueous, Arch. Ophth., 7, 538, 1932; 8, 9, 1932.
4. Magrane, William G.: Canine Glaucoma I—Methods of Diagnosis, J.A.V.M.A., 131, 311–314, 1957.
5. Lovekin, Louise G.: Primary Glaucoma in Dogs, J.A.V.M.A., 145, 1081–1091, 1964.
6. Magrane, William G.: Canine Glaucoma II—Primary Classification, J.A.V.M.A., 131, 372–374, 1957.
7. Magrane, William G.: Canine Glaucoma III—Secondary Classification, J.A.V.M.A., 131, 374–378, 1957.
8. Magrane, William G.: Thesis—Canine Glaucoma, Graduate School of Med., University of Pennsylvania, 1956.
9. Teng, C. C.: Glaucomatous Cupping, Am. J. Ophth., 58, 379–407, 1964.
10. Wright, J. G.: Clinical Case Records, Beaumont Hospital, Royal Veterinary College, 1937.
11. Formston, C.: Observations on Subluxation and Luxation of the Crystalline Lens in the Dog, J. Comp. Path. & Therap., 55, 168, 1945.
12. Magrane, William G.: Canine Glaucoma IV—Medical and Surgical Treatment, J.A.V.M.A., 131, 456–464, 1957.
13. Überreiter, Von Otto: Examination of the Eye and Eye Operations in Animals, *Advances in Veterinary Science*, Vol. 5, New York, Academic Press, Inc., p. 67, 1959.
14. Knight, Gordon: The Indications and Technique for Lens Extraction in the Dog, The Veterinary Record, 74, 1065–1069, 1962.
15. Meyer, S. J.: The Physiopathology and the Technique of Iridencleisis, Am. J. Ophth., 35, 78, 1952.

Chapter 10

DISEASES AND SURGERY OF THE LENS

Embryology, Anatomy and Physiology

10:1   Andersen and Shultz[1] have observed that the stages of lens development in the dog are similar to that of man. The dog embryo at twenty-three days is 5 mm long, and at this stage the lens pit is formed. At twenty-seven days (15 mm) a well-developed lens vesicle containing lenticular fibers is evident. It is not until the fetus is 24 to 25 mm long (mid-gestation) that the secondary lens fibers begin to form. These proliferate from the equator of the lens toward the posterior and central portions, forming the lens suture. It is during this stage of development that epithelial cells at the periphery of the lens secrete the lens capsule. Cells of secondary lens fibers remain at the equator as the so-called lens bow. This stage of lens development is of concern since inherited (congenital) cataract has its beginning as a capsular lens defect.

10:2   The crystalline lens is a transparent body suspended in the anterior portion of the eyeball between the aqueous and vitreous chambers. The depression in the anterior surface of the vitreous humor into which the lens is set is called the *patellar fossa*. Anteriorly the iris rests on the lens surface.

10:3   Prince's[2] measurements show that the lens is usually about 9 to 11.5 mm in diameter (most frequently about 9.5 mm) and 7 mm thick in the antero-posterior direction. Its volume is in the region of 0.5 cc. Its surfaces are more similarly curved than the lens in man which is biconvex in shape.

10:4   The lens is completely enclosed within an elastic *capsule* (anterior and posterior surfaces), which varies in thickness. The posterior capsular

187

thickness is seldom more than 7 per cent of the anterior thickness, the two thicknesses being 3.5 and 50 μ respectively. Unlike man, there is little variation in thickness in the anterior capsule.

10:5 The lens is held in position by its *suspensory ligament* (zonules). The zonular ligaments are numerous and dense. They connect with a narrow area of the lens capsule at its equator, but they travel widely in the opposite direction, covering the ciliary processes both posteriorly and anteriorly, and spreading backwards towards the retina.

10:6 The lens consists of a peripheral portion, the *cortex,* and a central part, the *nucleus.* The cortex is semi-solid and softer than the nucleus. In old age the entire lens is of the consistency of the nucleus and is hard and unyielding.

10:7 All the lens fibers are bound together with an amorphous medium which appears to be most noticeable just under the capsule and is a kind of anteroposterior central filament from which three other sheets project.[2] These are called *sutures* and they turn on themselves so they appear as an upright "Y" on one side of the lens, and an inverted "Y" on the other. These sheets of amorphous material receive and bind the ends of the lens fibers.

10:8 The lens is devoid of blood vessels except in fetal life, its nourishment being derived from the intraocular fluids. Being a living structure with definite metabolic needs, it must be supplied with nourishment, and the end products of metabolism must escape from it. These functions must be carried on without interfering in any way with the transparency of the lens.

10:9 The formation of new lens fibers takes place throughout life. As the formation of new lens fibers takes place, the older fibers are compressed and pushed in toward the center. This results in an increasing density of the lens from the surface to the center. The increasing density of the center, or nucleus, with increasing age is also the result of a loss of water, as well as compression of the lens fibers. If it were not for this process of sclerosis, the lens would soon grow to a size incommensurate with the eyeball. With this compensating sclerosis a dense, hard nucleus is formed.

10:10 Therefore, after about age five in the dog, when ablation of a cataractous lens is contemplated, it is important that the nucleus be removed in its entirety.[3] It cannot be broken up and expected to be absorbed by the aqueous humor, as is the case in the younger animal when "needling" of the lens, or surgical procedures of a like nature, will bring about absorption of any lens debris remaining in the anterior chamber. In addition, in a young lens the albuminoids are low, so it is possible to get absorption, whereas as the lens becomes older the albuminoids increase in quantity and absorption is rendered nearly impossible.

10:11 The function of the lens in man is to focus rays so that they form a perfect image on the retina. To accomplish this, the refractive power of the lens must change with the distance of the object (accommodation), and is produced by a change in shape of the lens.

10:12 In the dog this function of the lens becomes relatively unimportant. So far as focusing range of the lens is concerned, the dog has distinct limitations. The poor accommodation (ability to focus) is the result of a weak ciliary muscle and a firm, well-implanted lens within the eye (Par. 1:3).

Diseases

10:13   *Congenital anomalies* of the lens are few in type. Persistent remains of the hyaloid artery (embryological) may be seen occasionally with high magnification as a small dot on the posterior capsule with an attached strand hanging in the vitreous.

Cataract

10:14   A cataract is defined as any *opacity of the lens or of its capsule*.

10:15   Opacification of its fibers and alteration in water content are the only pathologic changes the lens can undergo, since it has no blood supply after birth. It cannot react to deleterious physical and chemical agents by an inflammatory or allergic process, as is true with other tissues. The transport of nutrients and waste products to and away from the lens takes place by an exchange between the lens substance and the aqueous humor. Any changes in the composition of the aqueous, or in its rate of formation, might be expected to influence the metabolism of the lens. Further, since the lens is enclosed in a capsule, changes in the permeability of this membrane are important in the maintenance of a normal metabolism. Loss of transparency (cataract formation) may then be a sequela to this disturbance in metabolism.

10:16   Numerous theories have been advanced as to the cause of cataract formation, but each form is probably due to interference with some specific physiochemical mechanism, this probably being different in each of the different types seen clinically. The loss of any one of these mechanisms is sufficient to produce opacification of lens fibers.

Varieties and Classification. Cataracts may be classified under two main divisions: developmental and degenerative.

10:17   1. *Developmental Cataracts.* The normal development of the lens fibers and epithelium has been affected during growth by heredity, nutritional, or inflammatory changes. This group includes *congenital* and *juvenile* cataracts.

10:18   True *congenital* cataracts are not commonly recorded. They may be first noticed by an observant owner as a peculiar reflection in the eye of a young puppy. The clinician, in conducting a complete physical examination in the puppy, may ascertain its presence. Or, it may be much later in life or never noted, depending upon the degree of opacity. Most congenital cataracts remain stationary for life and do not interfere, noticeable, with vision.

10:19   In examining 1200 dogs at the age of four weeks to eight years with the ophthalmoscope, Westhues[4] observed this type of cataract in 34 dogs in the form of a disc-shaped opacity in the posterior half of the lens. He also found the opacities to be stationary and concluded that they develop during fetal life or in the first days postnatum.

10:20   Szutter[5] found that these opacities do not extend from the anterior half of the lens to the posterior, but lie at the depth of the posterior lenticular star, *i.e.,* parallel to the equatorial plane of the lens. He feels they might be an abnormality acquired at some time during fetal life as a local loosening of the lenticular fibers with formation of fissures, which, in turn, results in the opacities. He describes congenital cataract as "being characterized by sharp contours, a silver-wire glittering, and visible in incident light."

10:21   Andersen and Shultz[1] believe this form of cataract may best be explained as a defect in the development of the secondary lens fibers, apparently as the result of incomplete lens capsular continuity.

10:22   We have noted that congenital lens opacities may disappear, remain stationary, or that eventually the remainder of the lens becomes opaque. Szutter,[5] too, reports of the transient nature.

10:23   Another form of stationary congenital cataract may be caused by persistent pupillary membrane (Par. 7:21). Persistent remnants of the membrane originate from the collarette and course in varying numbers toward the anterior surface of the lens (Fig. 122). In the area of insertion on the lens there is often a circumscribed opacity (anterior polar cataract) and pigmentation.

10:24   *Juvenile* cataracts are not uncommon, (Plate 10A) and it is with this group we need be most concerned. There is apparently a heredofamilial predisposition to complete lens opacity and blindness in a number of breeds. Whereas developmental cataract may afflict any individual within a breed, the fact remains that certain breeds and strains within breeds are prone to this affliction.

10:25   Early cataract development (one to six years of age) occurs most often in poodles, cocker spaniels, wirehair terriers, Boston terriers, miniature schnauzers and Afghan hounds. Breed popularity and geography will, of course, have a direct bearing on the number seen. Smythe[6] has seen the greatest percentage of cataracts, in proportion to the number of individuals, in the sealyham breed. When family backgrounds have been made available, it has often been ascertained that a parent or grandparent on either side also had early cataract.

10:26   *2. Degenerative Cataracts.* The normally developed lens substance loses its transparency as a result of degenerative changes from various causes. In this group are placed senile nuclear and cortical cataracts, diabetic cataracts, traumatic cataracts, radiation cataracts and cataract associated with systemic disease or poisoning (toxic cataract).

10:27   True *senile* cataract, with loss of vision, is not encountered nearly as often as is the juvenile type. A dog must live to a "ripe old age" before lens changes exert a demonstrable effect on vision. Rather, examination of most middle age to aged dogs reveals a bluish-grey haze back of the pupil which is often erroneously referred to as senile cataract.

10:28   In reality, this apparent loss of translucency is due to *nuclear sclerosis* (Par. 10:9). Because the lens fibers have increased in density some rays entering the lens are reflected back, giving the impression that a cataract is present. When ophthalmoscopy is used for the purpose of examining the lens (Par. 2:27) and fundus, it will be noted that, aside from the lens aberration, the fundus is quite clear to view.

10:29   *Diabetic cataracts.* The incidence of cataract development in diabetic dogs cannot be considered high. Diabetes, however, whether it is controlled or not, will predispose to cataract formation. In those instances, where the diagnosis has been made and the dog is under treatment, it may be concluded that sudden cataract development is due to the disease. But, it is axiomatic that if a middle age dog is presented with only a history of *rapid* cataract development and a sudden loss of vision, diabetes should be suspected. In the absence of the usual systemic clinical signs of diabetes, urine and blood sugar tests will confirm the suspicion. It is also noteworthy that juvenile cataracts usually develop earlier than middle age and seldom with "overnight" suddenness, and that senile cataracts are even slower and in very old age. This places diabetic cataract in a fairly distinctive age group.

10:30 *Traumatic* cataracts are known to occur as the result of a perforating wound of the lens capsule. Within a few hours to a few days after a perforating injury, the lens becomes cloudy from the absorption of aqueous. Soon the entire lens becomes opaque. Contusion cataract may not develop for many weeks after an injury.

10:31 *Radiation* induced cataracts must be considered rare in the dog.

10:32 *Toxic* cataract may result from circulation of disease toxins or poisons (*e.g.* naphthalene). Smythe[6] lists distemper-like diseases and uremias as possible causes.

10:33 *Secondary Cataract.* (Plate 10E) It is not uncommon for the lens to become gradually opaque in association with or following a complete retinal degeneration (Par. 11:59). This may occur at any age. I am unsure as to whether this type of cataract should be considered developmental or degenerative, so it is placed in a separate category.

10:34 Barnett[7] describes it thusly. "The first signs are usually of cortical cataract, frequently posterior, rarely anterior, sometimes both. The cataract often appears in the form of marks or lines on the faces of the lens and never completely obscures the lens in its early stages. These marks may take the form of a posterior polar cataract or, far more frequently, appear as lines crossing radially from the lens periphery towards its center. As development proceeds the lens substance becomes involved, taking on the appearance of a soft granular diffuse cataract. Later this cataract becomes dense and total and may show the typical "Y" suture marks on its anterior face. At this stage it is quite impossible to examine the retina and the cataract may be mistaken for a primary cataract suitable for operation. The absence of a pupillary reflex in the secondary cataract will distinguish it from a primary one obscuring a healthy retina, as however dense the cataract may be in these latter cases, a brisk pupillary reaction to light will be seen."

Stages of Cataract

10:35 1. *Incipient Stage* (Plate 10A and Fig. 151). The opacity most frequently begins as streaks or vacuoles extending from the nucleus. There is no noticeable loss of vision.

10:36 2. *Immature Stage* (Plate 10B). The lens becomes cloudy throughout with an actual increase in the total size of the lens. In this stage a "fundic reflex" will be still discernible and portions of the fundus may still be seen, though hazily. If both eyes are similarly involved, the dog will experience some difficulty in getting around.

10:37   3. *Mature Stage* (Plate 10C). In this stage the lens loses most of its fluid, shrinks somewhat, and becomes completely opaque. A "fundic reflex" cannot be discerned. In this stage the cataract is often referred to as being "ripe" since it can be extracted by extracapsular means without leaving much cortex behind. The dog becomes totally blind if both eyes are involved.

10:38   4. *Hypermature Stage* (Morgagnian cataract) (Plate 10D). A cataract may progress from the mature to the hypermature stage slowly or quite rapidly. The lens becomes still smaller in size, the cortex liquifies and may become milky or "speckled" in appearance. The nucleus sinks to the bottom of this fluid. There may be a return of vision (second sight) due to the "clearing" of the lens.

Symptoms and Diagnosis

10:39   Ordinarily a case is not presented for diagnosis until an owner notices that the dog is becoming a bit insecure, is missing a tossed ball, or occasionally hits a table leg. Or, the owner may attribute these changes in behavior to clumsiness until such time that the subject experiences real difficulty in getting around. Cataracts resulting in sudden loss of vision (Par.

10:29), on the other hand, will initiate a quick request for an examination.

10:40   As Knight[8] has indicated, "a remarkable feature of cataracts in dogs is the degree of vision retained in spite of their diffuse bilateral formation, providing the retinae are healthy. The lenses have to lose considerable transparency before vision is seriously impaired or lost."

10:41   Therefore, it becomes relatively simple to make a diagnosis of cataract by the method suggested (Par. 2:5 and 2:27). To determine the extent of lens involvement, dilatation of the pupil is necessary (Par. 3:31). A number of tests have been suggested[9] for the locating of opacities and the depth of opacities of the lens. The use of depth perception in the gross examination, and proper use of the ophthalmoscope obviates the need for employing these tests.

10:42   There are no inflammatory symptoms except when cataract is associated with intraocular disease (Par. 7:36) or with intumescence and secondary glaucoma (Par. 9:80). Hypermaturity may also provoke inflammatory symptoms (Par. 9:81).

10:43   *Predilection.* As has been noted in glaucoma (Par. 9:45), there

---

Plate 10.

A. Juvenile cataract. Incipient stage. Pupil dilatation is artificial. Note tapetal reflection through unaffected portions of the lens.

B. Juvenile cataract. Immature stage. Pupil dilatation is artificial. Lens opacity diffuse but a "fundic reflex" is still discernible.

C. Juvenile cataract. Mature stage. Pupil dilatation is artificial. Oblique view demonstrates shrunken, irregular, and dense white appearance of the lens.

D. Morgagnian cataract. Pupil pathologically dilated due to a secondary tension increase. Note tapetal reflection through the liquified cortex, and the nucleus settled on the bottom. The upper corneal vascularization is indicative of this toxic stage.

F. Final post operative appearance following a successful extracapsular cataract extraction. Note iridectomy above and absence of the capsule in that area. A tapetal reflection is present throughout in spite of the remaining capsular debris.

E. Cataract secondary to progressive retinal atrophy in the poodle. Pupil dilatation is pathological. Note tapetal reflection still visible and accentuation of the "Y" suture. Courtesy: Keith C. Barnett, Cambridge, England.

Plate 10

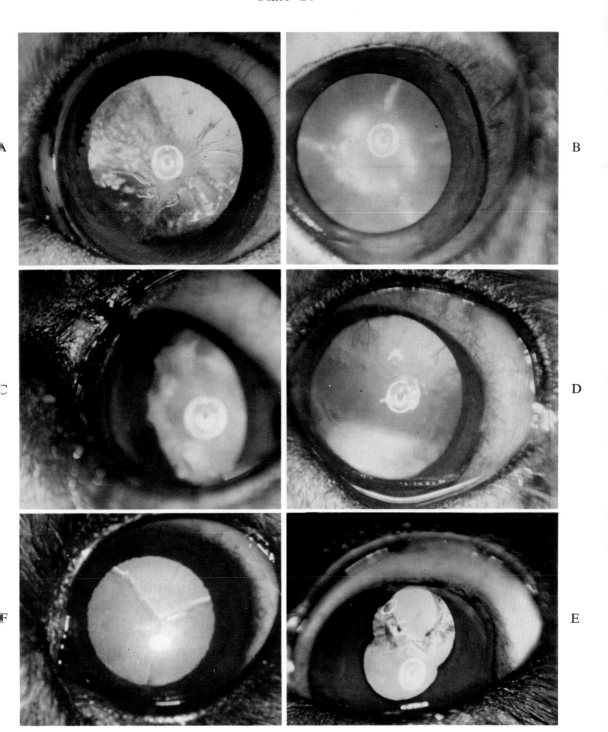

also seems to be a predilection for an initial left eye involvement in cataract. Usually the right eye exhibits an incipient stage, but it may well be several months before an opacity is noted in the second eye. In any event, with the exception of traumatic cataract, it is rare when the fellow eye is not soon similarly affected, with total blindness resulting.

Treatment

10:44   There is nothing known which significantly influences the progression of lens changes in cataract or prevents their formation. Claimed success for any treatment has been based on untrustworthy evidence or advanced by charlatans. Surgery is the only method for improving the vision in a blind or nearly blind eye. The need for surgery depends upon the vision of the fellow eye and the current status of the predominant eye.

Rationale[10]

10:45   Without some knowledge of the existing differences in the physiology and optics of man and dog, the veterinarian has assumed that, since strong, convex lenses and a proper refraction are requisites in order for man to obtain useful vision following a successful extraction, surely the dog will not benefit unless a corresponding refraction and an artificial lens also are used postoperatively.

10:46   This would be true, and would render the operation useless in the dog except that important optical differences do exist. In addition, the requirements for visual acuity do differ, and understandably so. The dog does not need the vision required for the reading of a newspaper, nor does it need to pursue an occupation dependent on reasonably good vision. It is important only that this restored vision will enable the animal to live out a normal life, free from the dangers and insecurity associated with bumping into furniture, being struck by a car, or stumbling up and down stairs.

10:47   Briefly, *aphakia,* or absence of the crystalline lens following surgical removal, is marked by a change in the focus of the dioptric system; or, simply, insufficient refracting power and loss of accommodation. The principal focus is considerably behind the retina, and convex lenses must be used, in man, to correct the ametropia. But here the differences between man and dog assume real meaning.

10:48   First, and of some importance, the dog accommodates poorly with a normal, intact lens. Therefore, absence of the lens is of little significance in this respect. Secondly, and of more importance, the dog is naturally myopic (nearsighted) and would not require nearly so powerful an artificial lens as man, even if one were "fitted" to him. Using arbitrary figures, man with an emmetropic eye (normal eye of 0 diopters) would require a plus 10 artificial lens to supplant the lens removed by surgery. By means of retinoscopy and ophthalmoscopy, it has been determined that the average dog is a minus 3 diopter myopic. Using these figures, then, it is apparent that even though an artificial lens were used, it would require one of only plus 7 strength, as opposed to the required plus 10 of man. Stated simply, the dog picks up three diopters of "vision" over man when both are subjected to lens removal.

10:49   Again, a knowledge of the dioptrics of the normal eye aids in the understanding of the true importance of the lens itself. In the optically normal eye the lens acts as, and can be compared with the fine adjustment of a microscope, adjusting the position of the image only in a minor way. The cornea itself carries most of the burden of placing the image on the retina. Actually, some highly myopic persons see clearly without glasses after a cataractous lens has been removed. With a normal lens in the eye they have too much focusing power. Thus, the more myopic a dog is before lens involvement with subsequent extraction the better it, too, will see.

10:50   There are, perhaps, other differences with which we are not familiar and which might well have a bearing on the fact that the blind dog sees so well following a successful cataract extraction. Almost unbelievable results have been achieved in a consequential number of dogs which were nearly or totally blind before undergoing surgery. Whereas the owner and I would have been happy to note return of ambulatory vision, many animals were, in addition, again able to run and play without any hesitancy. They were even able to follow and catch a bouncing ball.

10:51   Others[8, 9, 11–16] have agreed that cataract surgery in the dog is most feasible. Überreiter aptly states, "the poor results of early animal cataract surgery is no justification for rejecting cataract extractions today. Nor is there a need for the use of spectacles or intraocular lens implants."

10:52   It is interesting to note, also, that when, for the sake of satisfying my curiosity, two postoperative cases actually were refracted by retinoscopy and "fitted" with an appropriately ground contact lens by a specialist in this field, the animals wore and tolerated these lenses and did not object to their daily removal or reinsertion. This bit of investigation was still more gratifying, however, in that, although vision appeared to be improved some through use of the lenses, it was satisfactory enough without them to preclude the routine use of artificial lenses on practical and economical grounds.

General Considerations; Selection of Cases[17]

10:53   It is not the intent to leave the impression that results following surgery are 100 per cent, or that every blind animal with cataracts should be placed on the prospective operative list, or that even when good results are obtained they are to be expected at once. Neither can the results be expected to be constant in a series of the same breed or age group. Some animals will have better close vision, others better far vision, and many will have an adjustment period to pass through before a final evaluation can be made.

10:54   In removing the crystalline lens in cataract surgery, we have altered the lens system and the size of the image which falls upon the retina. When the signals thus elicited are transmitted to the brain and to consciousness, they are misinterpreted, especially as to localization. The conscious mind must relearn a skill and interpret the retinal stimuli on a new basis. Fortunately, this adjustment takes place rather rapidly in most instances, but then again "tincture of time" must be prescribed.

10:55   Although all of these considerations are important, they are of little consequence unless the proper preoperative preparation and evaluation of each case are carried out, and unless a good surgical technique is employed, with postoperative care receiving its just due. The optical and physiological differences discussed mean nothing if the operator is not prepared to devote an unusual amount of time to the perfection of one of the accepted techniques employed in human cataract surgery. There is no "short cut" to successful cataract surgery, and until this fact, well known to the ophthalmic surgeon, is accepted by his veterinary counterpart, he will be discouraged constantly by the results obtained. It is unfortunate that, for the most part, techniques previously described in veterinary literature have not fulfilled this criterion, and the reader has employed procedures which are too often doomed to failure even before they are attempted.

10:56 Age of the dog, degree of preoperative myopia, absence of complications, and other unexplained factors have a bearing on the degree of vision return. Failures cannot be attributed to the operation in principal, but rather to poor technique or improper selection of cases. A good basic knowledge of ophthalmology is essential to success. It is not sufficient simply to be an accomplished surgeon. An understanding of the macroscopic and microscopic anatomy, and the physiology of the eye, is the first requisite. In addition, a knowledge of ophthalmic pathology is a most important aid in the proper selection of cases. Some lens extractions, even though properly executed, are doomed to failure without this knowledge. It is of no use to remove the cataract from an eye in which the retina has been destroyed by glaucoma (Par. 9:35), progressive retinal atrophy (Par. 11:59), or diabetes (Par. 12:15). When the lens is so cloudy that the retina is invisible, it may become impossible to

diagnose rather extensive retinal disease, but every effort should be made to do so.

10:57 The steps which should precede endorsement of a cataract operation include: examination of the adnexa for infection, determination of tension of the eye by digital or instrumental tonometry, an urinalysis and a general physical examination in the middle aged and older patient, and above all a *check of the pupillary response to light stimuli*. The pupil must react promptly and normally. Interference or absence of this reflex is indicative of a retinopathy. Even in the presence of an apparently normal reflex, however, it is possible for the eye to be in the throes of a retinopathy which would preclude eventual success as regards return of vision. Unfortunately, in these instances, this determination cannot be made until after surgery. Then, by means of ophthalmoscopy, the retinal changes are evident and the reason for the failure of vision return is apparent.

10:58 Other considerations which are important to the degree of success achieved are: adequate practice surgery, a sufficient number of cases for perfection of a technique, and religiously adhering to the time-proven procedures of preoperative care, surgical technique, and postoperative care practiced by ophthalmologists in human medicine (Par. 3:94).

10:59 Those who have performed intraocular surgery almost invariably have wisely solicited the aid of an ophthalmologist for their initial attempts. It is then that both the veterinarian and the medical doctor learn that the dog's eye presents a more difficult surgical field than does the human eye. Proper exposure of the eye is sometimes difficult, the structures through which incisions must be made are tougher, more hemorrhage is encountered, and the lens itself is more firmly attached.

10:60   Cataract extraction is not usually performed unless both eyes are similarly involved and/or unless total, or imminent blindness is evident. On a number of occasions, I have operated one blind eye at the owner's request, but only if it was apparent that cataract was starting in the second eye. This routine offers the advantage of restoring vision to one eye as the second goes blind. Admittedly, however, the results are not as dramatic since the owner and patient are never exposed to the trials attending total blindess.

10:61   It is not necessary, as it was once advocated, to wait until a cataract is "ripe" (Par. 10:37). Conversely, it is often to the surgeon's advantage to remove the cataract before hypermaturity occurs (Par. 10:38). This often takes place rapidly and unbeknown to the owner and surgeon. The advantage to the patient and owner in performing surgery as soon as blindness ensues is apparent.

Surgery

10:62   The type of operation needed for removal of a cataract depends upon the consistency of the cataract (stage), the age of the patient, and the presence of intraocular complications such as adhesions.

10:63   The two methods of lens removal are:

1. *Extracapsular.* The anterior capsule of the lens is opened by means of a cystitome or capsule forceps and the lens content is expelled, leaving the posterior capsule and zonular attachments intact (Plate 10F).

2. *Intracapsular.* No opening is made in the lens capsule. The zonular attachments are severed and the lens is delivered enclosed within its capsule.

10:64   Variations employed with either the extracapsular or intracapsular extraction include:

(*a*) *combined* extraction—in which an iridectomy, including the pupillary border (sphincter), is performed (Plate 10F).

(*b*) *round pupil* extraction—in which one or more peripheral iridectomies or iridotomies, away from the sphincter, is performed.

(*c*) *simple* extraction—in which the extraction is performed without iridectomy or iridotomy.

10:65   There are, of course, advantages and disadvantages pertinent to the two methods and their variations. It remains for the surgeon to evaluate these procedures as they apply to the case at hand and as to his ability to execute the technique.

10:66   Extracapsular lens extraction is preferred in most instances. This is especially true in juvenile cataract surgery. It has proved the safest procedure because of the difficulty and danger attending the breaking of the tough lens attachments (zonules), and posterior vitreous attachment inherent to the young dog. Since loss of vitreous is one of the most important complications in cataract surgery, every effort is made to avoid this complication. The use of intraocular alpha-chymotrypsin to aid in the lysis of the zonules for the purpose of performing an intracapsular extraction has not been successful in the dog. This is not so much because zonular lysis fails to take place, but the posterior capsule of the lens is attached firmly to the face of the vitreous (Par. 11:3) and separation of the two (intracapsular extraction) will allow the escape of some portion of the vitreous.

10:67 Überreiter[9] is convinced, after large-scale comparative trials in the dog, that the extracapsular technique is far less dangerous. Vierheller[13] has found that the pressure required to tumble or express the lens from the eye within its capsule is often enough to create disastrous vitreous prolapse. Knight[8] attempts an intracapsular extraction, but confesses that in only a few instances has he been fortunate enough to find a hyaloid membrane intact after an uncomplicated total extraction. His results and percentage of success reported by this method are not encouraging.

10:68 Disadvantages of the extracapsular approach are: (1) broken down lens tissue in the eye which may result in various types and grades of inflammation. This condition has been attributed to an allergic reaction of the eye to the lens tissue; (2) the presence of capsular and lens debris in the pupillary area predisposes to iris adhesions with a small or occluded opening resulting.

10:69 These pupillary adhesions constitute the most vexing complication attending the extracapsular extraction. Mydriatics and cycloplegics, even when used early, frequently, and in high concentration, have been of questionable value in preventing occlusions when debris is present in appreciable amounts. However, in the young dog these complications occur infrequently if care is taken to keep debris and blood clots at a minimum. The performance of a combined extraction (Par. 10:64) is also of help in preventing pupil closure.

10:70 In my original series[17] it was concluded that results attending the iridectomy group versus the non-iridectomy group were about the same. Since that time a change in technique has produced more consistent results and an increased percentage of success. The iridectomy is now done with the electrocautery (Par. 7:81), thus facilitating the extraction, and eliminating the hemorrhage factor. Vierheller[13] performs a broad iridectomy, controlling all hemorrhage before proceeding to the extraction. Majilton[12] believes that an iridectomy is most important to success. Knight[8] is of the opinion that the iridectomy cannot be expected to serve a purpose in the dog. Roberts[14] avoids an iridectomy because it predisposes to a plastic iritis with a tendency toward synechiae.

10:71 Degenerative cataracts (senile and diabetic) may be extracted by the extracapsular method with good results. We have found, however, that any remaining lens debris in the older or diabetic patient creates far more intraocular reaction. To minimize this reaction it is now routine to make a subconjunctival steroid injection upon completing surgery, and to administer systemic steroids and antihistamines for one week postoperatively.

10:72 Due to the nature of the cataract (Par. 9:81), a hypermature lens should be removed by the intracapsular method whenever possible. If the capsule should rupture during extraction, it is important that its toxic content be irrigated from the anterior chamber and that steroids and antihistamines be used in the manner described (Par. 10:71).

10:73 The percentage of success could certainly be increased were an uncomplicated intracapsular extraction possible in every instance. The advantage of a clear pupil area and relative freedom from intraocular reaction and adhesions are apparent. But the disadvantage of possible vitreous prolapse into the anterior chamber, thereby producing multiple complications, is not to be taken lightly. In the older dog an intracapsular extraction becomes easier. In my original series[17] a 50 per cent success ratio was achieved in the senile group as opposed to 33 per cent in which extracapsular extraction was performed. Conversely, in the juvenile group 50 per cent success was achieved by the intracapsular route as opposed to 80 per cent in which an extracapsular extraction was performed.

10:74   Since this series[17] has been recorded, it has been evident that with each succeeding refinement incorporated into the operation the percentage of success has increased (in both age groups). I am also of the opinion that further research will make possible increased use of the intracapsular technique, with results approximating those achieved in human cataract surgery.

10:75   *Discission or needling* is mentioned only to condemn it as a method for correction of cataract. In the very young patient, with a soft cataract, the results may be encouraging. However, these cases are few in number, and it usually is impossible to ascertain the exact lens consistency on preoperative examination.

10:76   The operation consists of introducing a discission knife or knife-needle through the conjunctiva 1 to 2 mm from the limbus and then through the limbus into the capsule of the lens, making several cross cuts. The cortex may be broken by rotating the knife. The lens substance swells and some of it falls into the anterior chamber. Presumably the aqueous eventually absorbs

the lens content. Repeated "needling" may be needed to achieve this result.

10:77   Discissions can be followed by severe intraocular reaction or infection because of the large amount of lens matter left behind. Lens cortex is an ideal medium for the growth of organisms.[18] In many cases the source of this infection is the patient's own organisms.

10:78   Rapid and extensive swelling of the lens may also cause a secondary tension rise requiring immediate lens ablation. Iritis following discission is also a possibility.

The Operation

10:79   It is beyond the scope of this chapter to enumerate and describe all of the variations in technique employed by ophthalmic surgeons. A myriad of books and papers have been written on the subject of human cataract surgery and, as mentioned in the Preface, the interested reader should seek further knowledge in this specialized field by reference to these publications.

10:80   However, I will outline the steps of a technique applicable to the dog which has produced gratifying results. Also, instead of giving a complete discussion of operative complications which may preclude success, attention is drawn to important considerations which will prevent these complications.

Steps

10:81   The preoperative preparation of the patient, suitable operating area, positioning of the patient for surgery, instruments needed (with the exception of special ones), and anesthesia required are all enumerated in Chapter 3 —General Consideration for Eye Surgery.

10:82 1. *Canthotomy* (Par. 4:11) (Fig. 40). Elongation of the palpebral fissure is usually necessary in poodles, schnauzers, and wire-hair terriers. It is seldom required, for example, in cocker spaniels.

10:83 2. *Conjunctival flap* (Par. 9: 135). Advantages:

(*a*) As a solid tissue with Tenon's capsule, it is used as partial fixation support for preparing the groove and making the section.

(*b*) Acts as a mechanical covering for the wound, preventing further access of conjunctival secretions into the wound.

(*c*) Its continuity with the superficial cornea assists in sealing the lips of the wound and keeping them from separating.

(*d*) Prevents the epithelium from entering the anterior chamber.

(*e*) The exudate of plasma and fibrin found from severed conjunctival vessels binds or seals the wound completely. Infection is inhibited, repair promoted.

Disadvantages:

(*a*) The flap may tend to obstruct the surgeon's view of the chamber and act as a hindrance in making the section (easily overcome by holding the flap perpendicularly).

10:84 3. *Preliminary groove* (Par. 9:136). Preparation of the groove with the electroscalpel eliminates hemorrhage, presenting a clear, dry field for the placing of sutures. There has been no noticeable retardation in wound healing. Disadvantage—possibility of burning the conjunctival flap.

10:85 4. *Preplaced sutures* (Par. 9: 137). Four sutures are usually sufficient for the extracapsular extraction, five for the intracapsular method.

Advantages:

(*a*) Easier to place in the formed eye.

(*b*) Eliminates the hazard of manipulating the opened eye.

(*c*) Assures exact wound apposition when properly placed.

(*d*) Reduces incidence of shallow anterior chamber, iris prolapse and hyphema.[20]

Disadvantages:

(*a*) Increases the complexity of making and enlarging the section.

(*b*) Loops of suture to contend with (moistening with saline solution keeps loops in place).

10:86 Considerable research[19] has been conducted in the use of absorbable sutures for wound closure. Although chromic catgut continues to be advocated and used by many who are loath to the removing of non-absorbable sutures, the advantages of the latter are established. Non-absorbable sutures (silk, mersilene) produce less reaction, fewer wound infections, and can be counted on to hold the wound firmly closed until healing is well established. Catgut is stiff and more difficult to handle than silk; its knot is less secure and firm; and its tensile strength and absorption may vary so much with the degree of reaction as to render it unreliable for the important ten- to twelve-day period of wound healing. Mersilene offers the advantage of creating still less tissue reaction than silk, and it may be buried under a conjunctival flap, but it is, admittedly, harder to handle because of its kinkiness.

10:87 5. *Section* (Par. 9:139). The incision and enlargement of the incision throughout should be made in a moderately beveled manner. Beveled wounds have a valve-like action which prevents aqueous leakage. The bevel may be increased or decreased with corneal scis-

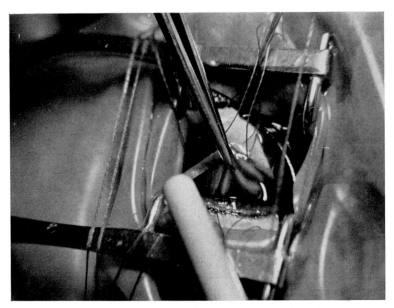

Fig. 141.   Iridectomy using the offset electroscalpel blade.

sors by tipping the blades. By making the section under the flap and on the scleral side as opposed to through clear corneas, scarring of the cornea is avoided. Very little hemorrhage accompanies a scleral incision, especially when the preliminary groove has been prepared with the electroscalpel.

10:88   6. *Iridectomy.* Whereas an iridectomy is not usually necessary for the extraction of a subluxated lens (Par. 9:140), it is of considerable help in cataract surgery. A combined extraction (Par. 10:64) allows for more working room for the extraction and is also of help in preventing pupil closure in the postoperative period.

10:89   Regardless of the mydriatic effect obtained in an eye preoperatively, there is a tendency towards pupil contraction following anesthesia and, especially after entering the anterior chamber. Use of a local anesthetic in the anterior chamber and the pre-warm irrigating solutions advocated by others

has not been of much help to me in preventing this miosis. The degree of contraction also differs considerably in individuals, making it almost mandatory that an iridectomy be performed in the patient whose pupil dilated poorly prior to surgery.

10:90   If the iridectomy is performed with the electroscalpel (Fig. 141) (moderate current setting), a clear, blood-free field may be obtained for the extraction.

10:91   7. *Extraction. Extracapsular—* several ways are used to open the lens. A cystitome may be used to tear the anterior capsule before removing some of it with forceps. In the dog, however, the capsule tends to "spring back" after being cut, making it difficult to find and extract. I prefer the use of capsule forceps (Fig. 142) for tearing and removing the anterior capsule. They are introduced into the section, rested lightly on the lens, spread for a distance of 3 to 5 mm, pressed gently but firmly against the lens, and closed so as to grasp a large portion of the capsule, while backward pressure is being exerted. Counter pressure, or a steadying effect on the lens, can be achieved by holding the capsule at the top of the lens with smooth capsule or tissue forceps held in the opposite hand. The capsule will often split at or near the vertical equator of the lens, thus most of the anterior capsule will be removed within the grasp of the forceps.

10:92 When the capsule has been opened and a sizeable "chunk" of anterior capsule has been removed, the lens content is ready to be expressed. In soft cataract (Par. 10:36) some of the cortex will begin to spill out. Sterile saline irrigation with a bulb and curved lacrimal needle worked into the lens will loosen and dislodge the content. Considerable irrigation is required to remove all of the cortex and nucleus in a soft cataract, and care must be taken that the irrigation process is slow and gentle to avoid endothelial damage (Par. 6:12). In mature cataract a lens loop is used to encompass the content just anterior to the intact posterior capsule. A forward and upward movement will bring the solid mass to the incision site. Subsequent irrigation is needed to remove residual cortex. But overzealousness on the part of the surgeon to remove the last bit of cortex may lead to complications. It is best to permit some cortex to absorb rather than use too much force and thus increase the danger of vitreous loss or permanent damage to the endothelium.[22] When a fundic reflex is discernible and/or a fairly clear black pupil is established, the lens content removal can be considered complete.

10.93 *Intracapsular*—Traction with pressure is used to express the lens in its capsule. "Tumbling," "sliding," and suction (erisophake), with stripping of the zonules as needed, are methods commonly employed. In the dog, rupture of the capsule occurs rather frequently, thus leading to an extracapsular extraction.

10:94 8. *Closure.* The preplaced sutures are drawn up. All lens debris should be cleared from the lips of the wound before the ties are made. A triple tie is recommended. Following the first tie the wound opposition should be checked before securing the knot. This applies to each of the sutures. Up to ¼ cc of 1 to 1000 adrenalin is floated into the anterior chamber before the final tie is made. This tends to aid in producing the desired postoperative mydriasis. Following closure, an air bubble is injected between sutures with the dry irrigation bulb and needle. This reforms the anterior chamber immediately, thus preventing the formation of

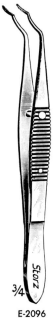

E-2096

Fig. 142. Extracapsular capsule forceps.

anterior synechia. Reforming the anterior chamber with air also serves to test the integrity of the closure.

10:95   Tenon's capsule and the conjunctiva are replaced and sutured with 5–0 or 6–0 chromic catgut, depending on the tissue thickness. Used Greishaber needles work nicely for this purpose. The two layers may be sutured separately or together with a continuous running suture tied on both ends. A drop of 4 per cent atropine and an antibiotic is instilled, the canthotomy wound is closed, a single mattress suture is placed to close the lids (Fig. 139), and a bandage is applied (Par. 3:81) (Fig. 31).

10:96   *Postoperative Care.* This is similar to that recommended following glaucoma surgery (Par. 9:143). Bandaging is important for the reasons elicited (Par. 3:80). Dressings may be changed daily or on alternate days with instillation of atropine and the antibiotic used following surgery. Bandaging may be discontinued after four or five days. I have run a series in which comparisons were made between bandaged and unbandaged eyes. Those eyes bandaged for four to six days "quieted" down and presented fewer complications than the unbandaged eyes.

10:97   The lid suture is removed a week following surgery. Atropine and a steroid-antibiotic are used several times a day and for as long as one month postoperatively. The corneoscleral sutures are never removed before the twelfth postoperative day (Par. 9:144). The conjunctival suture is left to absorb.

10:98   Careful handling of the patient, freedom of excitement, and the use of protective collars (Fig. 140) for at least the first week are important during hospitalization. I am not in ac-

cord with the practice of sending a cataract case home several days after surgery, even if the patient could be kept quiet at home. Daily checks are important for the first two weeks to ascertain possible complications which would go unnoticed by the owner.

10:99   *Postoperative Complications.* The most frequent complication following an extracapsular extraction will be formation of pupillary adhesions (Par. 10:68). Adhesions are unimportant, however, provided the opening is sufficient for light to reach the retina and the aqueous circulation is free. Whereas a large pupil free of adhesions is always desirable, a small pupil and a clear opening to the fundus is often sufficient to allow for useful, regained vision.

10:100   The other major complications of cataract surgery, both early and late, *e.g.,* vitreous prolapse, iris prolapse, corneal opacity, hemorrhage, iritis and infection, are infrequently encountered if the aforementioned precautions are taken and a proven technique is perfected.

Dislocation of the Lens
(Plate 9B and C)

10:101   Dislocation of the lens may occur as a result of injury, from a hereditary predisposition, or to a combination of the two. Dislocation may be partial (subluxated) or complete (luxated).

10:102   Subluxation may consist of a tilting of one edge of the lens or of displacement to a superior, inferior, nasal (medial), temporal (lateral), or anterior position (Figs 143, 144 and 145). Luxation occurs when the ligamentous attachment of the lens is completely disrupted and when it has vacated the patellar fossa (Par. 10:2).

The lens is then usually displaced anteriorly into the anterior chamber in front of the iris (Fig. 146) or posteriorly into the vitreous.

10:103 Traumatic dislocation is generally the result of a blow upon the eye or it may occur following rupture of a corneal ulcer and sudden loss of the anterior chamber. By far the most important cause of lens dislocation in the dog is genetic instability in the suspensory apparatus (Par. 9:60).

10:104 *Clinical Signs.* These have been described in detail previously (Par. 9:65–9:68). Briefly, again, the early signs include: watery, sensitive, sometimes painful eye, iridodenesis (maybe only sign), inhibition of pupil reflex, corneal haze, scleral injection, and increased tension. The late signs include: the aphakic crescent (Plate 9B), in which an area of increased light reflex in a part of the pupil area is evi-

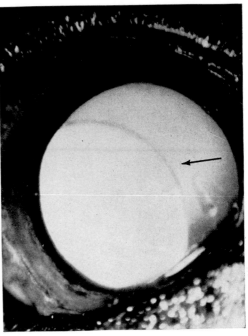

Fig. 144. Subluxation of the lens to the temporal position.

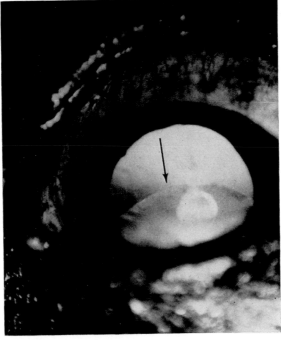

Fig. 143. Subluxation of the lens to the inferior position. Lens is becoming cataractous. Note congestion of conjunctival vessels and dilatation of pupil (secondary glaucoma).

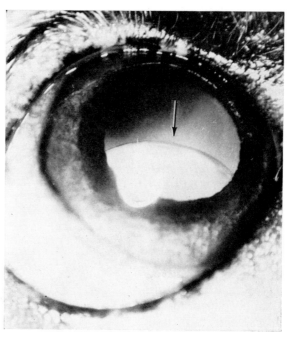

Fig. 145. Subluxation of the lens to the inferior position. Note near normal pupil and absence of congestive signs of secondary glaucoma.

dent (denoting displacement of the lens from that area), interstitial keratitis, and buphthalmos. Loss of vision will be present on the affected side or sides.

10:105   When the lens luxates completely into the anterior chamber or into the vitreous, the tension may return to normal with alleviation of the inflammatory symptoms. The completely dislocated lens soon becomes opaque (Fig. 147) and is then easily seen, regardless of its position.

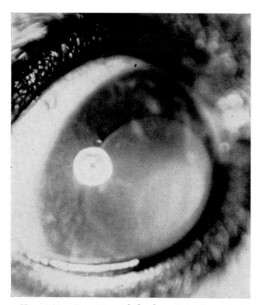

Fig. 146. Luxation of the lens into the anterior chamber with adhesion to the corneal endothelium.

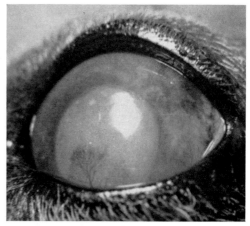

Fig. 147. Luxation of the lens into the anterior chamber. Note opaqueness of lens and superficial vascularization of the cornea.

10:106   Formston[23] summarizes the diagnostic features of lens displacement as follows:

(1) increased intraocular tension associated in its train with distension of the eyeball and scleral conjunctival congestion.

(2) a dilated pupil, an iris which reacts sluggishly to light, iridodenesis.

(3) a zone of pupillary aphakia with the edge of the lens partly or wholly visible.

10:107   *Breed incidence* and age (Par. 9:59) are important considerations to the establishment of a diagnosis when the clinical signs are not immediately discernible or prominent.

10:108   *Treatment.* The medical and surgical treatment of lens displacement has been discussed (Chapter 9). In summary, it is imperative that an early diagnosis be made if vision in an eye or eyes is to be retained by medical or surgical means.

10:109   *Prevention.* Involvement of the second eye in the heredofamilial type of lens displacement can be expected, therefore at least an effort should be made to prevent its occurrence. We caution owners to discontinue throwing balls, to discourage violent exercise, and not to allow the patient to pull hard on collar and lead. Daily use of a miotic that will keep the pupil in a partial state of miosis is sometimes helpful. This allows for additional support of the iris to the lens upon which it rests. The owner is asked to present the animal immediately at the first sign of irritative symptoms in the "good" eye.

References

1. Andersen, A. C. and Shultz, F. T.: Inherited (congenital) Cataract in the Dog, Am. J. Path., *34*, 965–975, 1958.
2. Prince, Jack H., Diesem, Charles D., Eglitis, Irma and Ruskell, Gordon L.: *Anatomy and Histology of the Eye and Orbit in Domestic Animals*, Springfield, Charles C Thomas, p. 82, 1960.
3. Magrane, William G.: Ocular Physiology–Clinical Application, No. Am. Vet., *36*, 563, 1955.
4. Westhues, M.: Arch. Tierheik, *54*, 32–83, 1926.
5. Szutter, L.: Ophthalmoskopische Und Lupenspielgelunter-suchungen An Neugeborenen Haustieren. II, Acta Veterinaria, Academiae Scientiarum Hungaricae, *11*, issue 2, 1961.
6. Smythe, R. H.: *Veterinary Ophthalmology*, London, Bailliere Tindall & Cox, 1956.
7. Barnett, K. C.: Hereditary Retinal Atrophy in the Poodle, The Vet. Record, *74*, 673, 1962.
8. Knight, Gordon C.: Canine Intraocular Surgery, The Vet. Record, *72*, 644, 1960.
9. Überreiter, Von Otto: Examination of the Eye and Eye Operations in Animals, *Advances in Veterinary Science*, Vol. 5, New York, Academic Press, Inc., 1959.
10. Magrane, William G.: Rationale of Cataract Surgery, No. Am. Vet., *35*, 759, 1954.
11. Greaud, R.: *Contribution au Traitement Chirurgical de la Cataracte Chez le Chien*, Paris, Imp. R. Foulon, 1950.
12. Majilton, E. A.: *Early Surgery for Cataracts*, Gaines Vet. Symp. Proc., New York, Gaines Dog Research Center, 1958.
13. Vierheller, Ralph C.: Canine Cataract Surgery, Vet. Med., *52*, 487, 1957.
14. Roberts, S. R.: Personal Communication, 1960.
15. Jensen, Harlen: Cataract–*Current Veterinary Therapy*, Philadelphia, W. B. Saunders Co., 1964–1965.
16. Custer, M.: Cataract Surgery, Proc. Am. Soc. Vet. Ophth., Chicago, 1964.
17. Magrane, William G.: Cataract Extraction: An Evaluation of 104 Cases, J. Sm. An. Pract., *1*, 163–168, 1961.
18. Fasanella, R. M.: *Modern Advances in Cataract Surgery*, Philadelphia, J. P. Lippincott Co., 1963.
19. Roper, K. L.: *The Cataract Operation–A Study of Details*, Manual Am. Acad. Ophth. & Otol., 1961.
20. Singh, D.: Pre-placed versus Post-placed Corneo-scleral Sutures in Cataract Surgery, Brit. J. Ophth., *47*, 116–122, 1963.
21. Spaeth, Edmund B.: *Principles and Practice of Ophthalmic Surgery*, 4th ed., Philadelphia, Lea & Febiger, 1948.
22. Weiner, Meyer and Scheie, Harold: *Surgery of the Eye*, 3rd ed., New York, Grune & Stratton, 1952.
23. Formston, C.: Observations on Subluxation and Luxation of the Crystalline Lens in the Dog, J. Comp. Path. & Therap., *55*, 180, 1945.

Chapter 11

DISEASES OF THE VITREOUS, RETINA AND OPTIC NERVE

Vitreous

11:1   *Anatomy.* The vitreous is a transparent, colorless, jelly-like mass filling the chamber of the eye behind the lens. It is attached to the pars plana of the ciliary body and to the optic nerve. The vitreous has no blood vessels, but receives its nourishment from the surrounding tissues, the choroid, ciliary body and retina. Its chemical composition is very similar to that of the aqueous humor with the exception of two proteins peculiar to the vitreous humor, mucoid and vitrein (which causes it to "jell-up").[1] One of the principal functions of the vitreous is to hold the retina smoothly in place.

11:2   The outer surface of the vitreous presents a thin condensation, the so-called *"hyaloid" membrane,* which serves to contain the vitreous and separate it from the posterior aqueous chamber. Recent electromicroscopy studies[2] of the human vitreous showed that the framework of the vitreous body consisted of interconnecting laminar aggregates formed by filaments. Anteriorly these filaments ended abruptly in an interwoven net to form the *face* or anterior border layer. No specialized limiting membrane that could be called a hyaloid membrane was observed. Thus, it is not clear as to what this membrane should be called.

11:3   In any event, the lens is cradled on this anterior condensation of the vitreous in what is known as the patellar fossa (Par. 10:2). In the dog the lens is somewhat firmly attached to this "face of the vitreous" (Par. 10:66).

When the lens has been removed, the normal anterior membrane is pressed forward by the vitreous. This membrane then becomes more opaque, increases in tensile strength, and pushes the vitreous back, forming a retaining wall between it and the aqueous. I have repeatedly observed this phenomenon following removal of a displaced lens. In spite of the rupture of this anterior limiting membrane, a second condensation takes place which serves to retain the vitreous.

Diseases of the Vitreous

11:4   Affections of the vitreous include: (1) degenerations; (2) opacities; and (3) abscesses.

11:5   *Synchysis scintillans* (fluidity of the vitreous) is an alteration in consistency occurring as a senile change (degeneration) or, secondarily, to disease of its neighboring parts, the choroid, ciliary body and retina. The vitreous becomes fluid and cholesterol crystals are present. These crystals move as a shower of glittering particles on quick movement of the globe, but settle down to the floor of the vitreous chamber after movement has stopped.[3] I[4] have encountered it in dogs from middle to old age, sometimes without any accompanying lens involvement, but in others with cataractous changes beginning. With movement of the eyeball, synchysis scintillans can be likened in appearance to the snow-filled, crystal-ball paperweight when it is turned end for end. Vision is not always appreciably impaired, but with the condition there is a predisposition to detachment of the retina, often diminished tension in the eyeball, and more likelihood of lens subluxation. Loss of vitreous would be almost a certainty were an intraocular operation performed.

11:6   *Asteroid Hyalitis* (Fig. 148) is characterized by minute solid bodies *suspended* in a substantially normal vitreous. These bodies are of different sizes and shapes with no orderly arrangement. They are seen to move upon motion of the head, but return to their original position in the vitreous.

11:7   The condition does not appear to cause reduced visual acuity or other symptoms in the dog and will usually go unnoticed unless the eye is examined

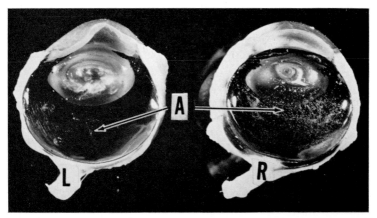

Fig. 148.   Asteroid hyalitis. Gross specimens of eyes (with calottes removed). Asteroid bodies (A) are numerous in right eye (R). Few are seen in the left eye (L). (Courtesy of Dr. Lionel Rubin, Philadelphia, Pa.)

for some other reason. It does appear far more frequently than does synchysis, and can be expected to be seen from middle age on. In one series of 300 dogs (beagles) between the ages of eight and ten, a 10 per cent incidence was noted (one or both eyes).

11:8   Rubin[5] examined the vitreous bodies of some representative cases of asteroid hyalitis and found them grossly normal. Tests also showed that the asteroid bodies were composed of a calcium lipid complex, similar chemically to that of man.

11:9   *Opacities* of the vitreous are not uncommon. They may occur as a consequence of the changes mentioned (synchysis, asteroid hyalitis), but usually they are the result of disease or of hemorrhages from the neighboring structures. A cloudy haziness often accompanies or follows uveitis (Par. 7:36). Hemorrhage into the vitreous may be total or may occur in strands. Vision will generally be affected. A diagnosis is made with the ophthalmoscope or pen-light held at a distance (Par. 2:27). For a detailed study the ophthalmoscope is used at the proper setting (Fig. 24).

11:10   Determining the cause of an intravitreal hemorrhage is often difficult. Contusion or perforating injury must certainly be considered. Certain systemic disorders (Chapter 12) may be held responsible. Strands of blood can be seen in the vitreous associated with retinal detachment. The vitreous may also contain blood when a hemorrhage into the anterior chamber is noted, but this cannot be verified unless the anterior chamber clears. Hemorrhage into the vitreous and anterior chambers has been noted following lens removal for absolute glaucoma. In these

cases it is thought that capillary permeability is increased as a consequence of the sudden lowering of tension to a state of hypotony.

11:11   Regardless of cause, the blood may be absorbed completely. If absorption does not occur, there is danger of organization and proliferation of the clot with the risk of a subsequent detachment of the retina.

11:12   *Treatment* consists of giving attention to any possible predisposing systemic affection and administering medication to increase coagulability of the blood and to decrease capillary permeability (Par. 3:88). I have enjoyed fair success by prescribing C.V.P. with K* and Adrenosen (2.5 mg)** for oral use. The average 25 pound dog is given one tablet of each twice a day. The use of systemic enzymes (Par. 3:67) and long term iodide therapy is helpful in promoting absorption of the clot.

11:13   *Abscess of the vitreous* denotes suppurative endophthalmitis in which the exudate remains confined to the vitreous (Par. 7:54). Treatment is that recommended for endophthalmitis (Par. 7:56).

Retina

11:14   *Anatomy.* The retina is a thin, delicate, transparent membrane which is really an invaginated extension of the brain to which it is connected by the optic nerve and its ramifications (Par. 1:9) (Fig. 3). The retina extends forward to the ciliary body, terminating at the *ora serrata* where it becomes continuous with the epithelium over the inner surface of the ciliary body. It is loosely attached to the choroid except at the ora serrata and in the optic disc

* U.S. Vitamin Corp.
** Massengil, Bristol, Tennessee.

area, thus, in detachment of the retina the membrane usually retains its hold at these two points. The retina is held in contact with the choroid by the pressure of the vitreous (Par. 11:1).

11:15   The retina of the dog is about 0.24 mm thick where there is a tapetum behind it, but tapers to 0.12 mm at the periphery, the dimensions being shared by all of its 10 layers.[6] Two forms of light-sensitive cells are found in the layers of the retina; *rods* which are exceedingly sensitive and are used for vision in low illumination and at night; and, *cones* which function at higher levels of illumination. Of these retinal receptors the rods predominate, the cones comprising little more than 5 per cent of the total receptors (Par. 1:4). There is no part of the retina actually free of rods in the dog as there is in man. There is, however, an area of greatest sensitivity, an area centralis (Par. 2:57) about 3 mm lateral to the optic nerve. It can be recognized by its freedom from large blood vessels and this is the area in which sharpest vision and discrimination is enjoyed. Prince[6] prefers to use the term "Macula" for this area because it relates this area to the terminology used for a similar area in the human eye; whereas, "area centralis" only denotes its position, not its function.

11:16   The retina is richly vascular, receiving a direct blood supply from main arteries or a cilioretinal network. Many microscopic capillaries are present within some of its layers. There are never less than four, and frequently as many as eight large vessels leaving the head of the optic nerve. These bifurcate freely, and together with several smaller ones which leave the optic nerve in radiating directions, they serve the whole retina, providing a rich capillary network right to the periphery.[6]

11:17   The ophthalmoscopic appearance of the background (fundus) and distribution of the retinal vessels are given in Chapter 2 (Par. 2:53 through 2:61).

Diseases of the Retina

11:18   *Affections of the retina* may be divided into: (1) congenital anomalies; (2) injury; (3) circulatory disturbances; (4) inflammation; (5) detachment; (6) tumor; and, (7) degenerations.

11:19   *Congenital anomalies* are uncommonly observed. A congenital hypoplasia of the optic nerve and retina in collie puppies, with blindness, has been described by Saunders.[7] In his series the vasculature of the retina appeared grossly normal but on histopathological examination it was apparent that the ganglion cell layer was involved. Our findings in several similar cases of near or total blindness included: (1) a collie with microphthalmia, lens opacities, and no visible retinal blood supply or optic disc; (2) collie pup with microphthalmia, congenital posterior cataract, observable choroidal and retinal circulation but no definite disc; and, (3) a minature poodle puppy in which the retinal vessels appeared intact but discs could not be discerned. An optic nerve hypoplasia was confirmed by necropsy in all three.

11:20   A congenital posterior ectasia of the sclera (Par. 11:69) will, in turn, result in degenerative changes in the retina with detachment and intraocular hemorrhage as common sequelae.[8] We have observed congenital retinal detachment in both the collie and Bedlington terrier breeds. Rubin[9] reported detachment in the Bedlington breed. These cases exhibited near or total blindness, the eyes were small in relation to the size of the palpebral fissure, cicatricial entropions were present, and the retinas were completely detached except at the ora serrata and optic disc. On histopathological examination an important additional finding was the lack of an inner retinal layer in the central portion of the retina and a diminished outer layer of rod and cone cells. Congenital cataract of varying degree was also noted in the eyes examined.

11:21   Rubin[10] also describes coloboma of the choroid in a coonhound in which the veins draining into and arteries emanating from the optic disc coursed around the crater of the coloboma, and small vessels, branches of the major retinal vasculature, dipped into the ectatic area. Histologically, the retina was completely disorganized in the depths of the ectatic area.

11:22   *Injury* of the retina may occur as the result of contusion of the eyeball. There is usually impaired vision, and a milky edema of the retina and hemorrhages within the layers will often be discernible. Treatment consists of rest, instillation of atropine, and systemic enzymes (Par. 3:67).

11:23   A transient blindness may result from injurious exposure of a dog's eyes to sunlight reflected from snow (snowblindness). This type of photoretinitis has been observed primarily in out-of-doors farm dogs exposed to rather long periods of brilliant sunlight and heavy snow cover. An accompanying conjunctival chemosis and catarrhal discharge (Par. 5:30) may be noted. The symptoms will disappear upon change of environment.

11:24   *Circulatory disturbances* of the retina, while common to man, are seldom encountered in the dog. Catcott[11] concludes, "the fact that retinal vascular lesions are seldom observed and are difficult to produce in the dog is attributed to the resistance of this species to vascular hypertension." However, it must be presumed that cyanosis, anemia, and hemorrhages of the retina occur as the result of systemic disease, but go unnoticed by the clinician unless subjective symptoms of impaired vision are prominent. Hemorrhages of the retina do occur as the result of septicemia, leptospiral infections, diabetes, heart conditions, poisoning, and in terminal nephritis (uremia).

11:25   *Inflammation* is seldom limited to the retina but is commonly associated with disease of the choroid or

---

Plate 11

A. Partial, funnel detachment of the retina originating from the optic disc area. Courtesy: Dr. R. Trueman. Philadelphia, Pa.

B. Complete retinal detachment (gross photograph). Note vessels within the retinal folds behind the dilated pupil. Retina lies near the posterior surface of the lens.

C. Advanced retinal degeneration. Note absence of nearly all retinal vessels. Courtesy: Dr. William Gay, Washington, D. C.

D. Retinal atrophy permitting visualization of the underlying choroidal circulation (lower fundus). Courtesy: F. Lescure, de l' Ecole Nationale Vétérinaire de Toulouse.

E. Congenital excavation of the optic disc (scleral ectasia) in the collie. Ectatic area most pronounced 11:00 to 4:00 o'clock. Courtesy: Dr. Leon Saunders, Philadelphia, Pa.

F. Intraocular hemorrhage associated with the collie disc anomaly.

G. Swollen optic disc with edema of the adjacent retina (neuroretinitis).

H. Exposed choroidal circulation as a consequence of absence of the tapetum. Vision normal. Note retinal vessels overlying the choroidal circulation and blending of the optic disc into the surrounding area.

Plate 11

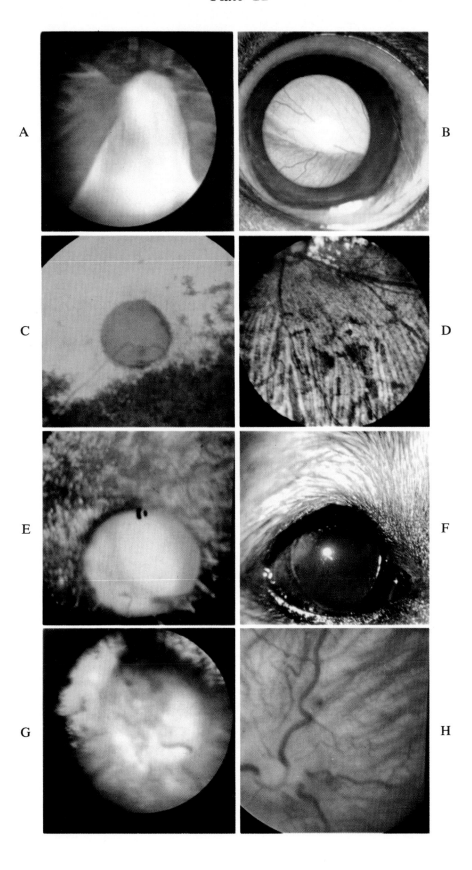

uveal tract (Par. 7:36). Because of the diffuse clouding of the ocular media, the changes in the retina are not usually apparent until the associated inflammation subsides. These changes include atrophy of the retina, allowing the choroidal vessels to become visible, with the presence of "eroded" areas and pigment migration throughout.

11:26 *Detachment* of the retina (Plate 11A and B) is a separation of the retina from the choroid. It may be partial or complete (except where it is attached at the ora serrata and optic disc) (Par. 11:14), and may affect one or both eyes. It may be congenital in origin (Par. 11:20) or may be due to disease or injury.

11:27 Roberts[12] divides retinal detachment into three principal groups and concludes that the pathogenesis and pathologic characteristics of detachment in the dog does not differ greatly from that of man.

11:28 1. *Forces Which Push the Retina Away from the Underlying Pigment Epithelium.* In chorioretinitis, subretinal exudates may be produced as a response by the tissues to infective agents. These exudates accumulate between the retina and pigment epithelium causing detachment of the area involved.

11:29 Parasites such as filaria may produce detachment by mechanical means, but mainly from the exudative reaction on neighboring tissues.

11:30 Neoplasia of the uveal tract (Par. 7:62) may cause detachment because of the intrusion of the neoplastic tissue between the two layers.

11:31 2. *Forces Which Pull the Retina Forward.* In intraocular infection, inflammatory exudates undergo contrac-tion in the cicatricial stage, and fibrovascular membranes develop which exert traction anteriorly on the ciliary body or retina, resulting in detachment. Intraocular blood clots may also organize, proliferate and produce strands which pull on and cause detachment of the retina (Par. 11:11).

11:32 Retinal detachment may also occur following vitreous loss from surgery or perforating injuries of the globe. Without support from solid vitreous (Par. 11:1), the retina is predisposed to detachment.

11:33 Detachment is seen after lens displacement, especially when the lens is deviated posteriorly toward the ciliary body, or into the vitreous cavity. Production of a cyclitis or vitreitis ensues with formation of membranes which pull the retina anteriorly.

11:34 3. *Retinal Tears and Cysts.* Tears in the retina or rupture of retinal cysts will allow fluid or vitreous to reach the subretinal area. In old dogs, especially those with retinal atrophy, small cysts may be seen close to the ora serrata or on the central parts of the retina.

11:35 *Clinical Signs of Detachment.* Unless or until a loss of vision is apparent, a dog will not be presented for examination. Small detachments do not markedly impair vision and thus will go unnoticed. The dog is presented only when the detachment progresses, or when a sudden, complete detachment occurs. Opacities of the ocular media may make it difficult or impossible to diagnose detachment.

11:36 In retinal detachment, the eye usually becomes hypotensive, and on gross examination (Par. 2:5) the pupillary response to light stimuli may be

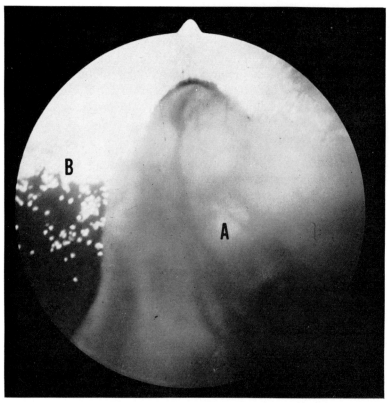

Fig. 149.   Retinal detachment (A) and retinal degeneration. Note absence of vessels in area not detached (B). Courtesy of Keith C. Barnett, Cambridge, England.

incomplete or absent. During this part of the examination, a detachment may be noted if it is extensive and central (Plate 11B).

11:37   The ophthalmoscopic appearance differs from case to case. The detached portion usually appears gray and silvery. This part may undulate or wave with movement of the eye. A detached portion may be seen as a billowing "cumulus cloud-like" mass which usually has a sharply defined edge on to the normal fundus. The retinal vessels are tortuous and can be seen to run up and down in the "hills and valleys." They may disappear beneath folds of detached retina. The ophthalmoscope setting must be changed constantly during the examination in order to visualize clearly the normal and abnormal zones (Par. 2:38).

11:38   Following retinal detachment a progressive atrophy takes place with eventual obliteration of all normal retinal architecture (Fig. 149). Late changes may include secondary cataract (Par. 10:33), uveitis, secondary glaucoma or phthisis bulbi.

11:39   *Treatment.* In man, early operative treatment is essential to success. These procedures include: perforating diathermy; electrolysis; surface coagulation; scleral resection; photocauterization; and, vulcanizing by cryo (freezing) methods. Because of the extent of the lesion in the dog, when first presented, and the special skills and equipment required, surgical correction is seldom possible.

11:40 However, we have experienced success in the medical treatment of obscure spontaneous detachment with sudden blindness. In these instances, a high therapeutic regimen of ACTH, Diuril,* and Chymar** resulted in absorption of the subretinal fluid, with reattachment and return of vision. Treatment with these products should be continued for ten to fourteen days before a hopeless prognosis is given.

11:41 The ACTH is repeated at forty-eight-hour intervals. The Chymar injections are given at twelve-hour intervals for five to seven days, after which the oral form may be used. The Diuril tablets are given at twelve-hour intervals. Rest and confinement is believed to be important to recovery.

11:42 *Tumors* of the retina will usually occur secondarily to uveal tract neoplasia (Par. 7:62). Grice and Hutchison[13] described a retinoblastoma, a congenital malignant tumor arising from the nuclear layers of the retina.

Degenerations (Plate 11C and D)

11:43 The most common affection of the retina is degeneration in its varying forms. Generally, we recognize two types of retinal atrophy: (1) the *hereditary* form; and, (2) degeneration as a sequela to *systemic* disease (distemper) (Par. 12:24), chorioretinitis (Par. 7:36), and deficiencies (Par. 3:58).

11:44 The hereditary form of progressive retinal atrophy has been reported in the literature as occurring in primarily the hunting breeds: the Gordon setter,[14] Irish setter,[15] Labrador retriever,[16] poodle,[17] English setter, pointer, Elkhound, springer spaniel, beagle, and cocker spaniel. But scattered cases of what appeared to be true hereditary, bilateral progressive retinal atrophy has been encountered in other breeds and in dogs of mixed breeding.[18]

11:45 In order to differentiate this form of retinal degeneration from that which may be the sequela to systemic disease, the following diagnostic criteria is suggested: (1) one owner possession since early puppyhood; (2) no history of previous illness of any importance; (3) loss of vision noted to be gradual by the owner; (4) no accompanying neurologic signs; and, (5) owner aware of "increased tapetal reflectivity" for some time.

11:46 In contrast, the retinopathy associated with or following distemper is diagnosed on a basis of: (1) history; (2) sudden blindness; and, (3) absence of prominent ophthalmoscopic findings. Parry[19] has concluded that the dog distemper virus can cause serious damage to the dog retina, either during the acute phases of the disease, or as a delayed sequela to the infection with a chronic generalized primary retinopathy which may develop slowly one to two years after the primary infection. He has reported[20] cases also of generalized progressive atrophy of uncertain etiology which are very similar to hereditary atrophy but with an onset later in life.

11:47 Thus, because of the difficulty in eliciting accurate histories, the possibility of virus infections hastening an existing predisposition to atrophic changes, and the further possibility that gradual loss of vision, or systemic and local diseases influencing vision may have gone unnoticed, it always will re-

---

* Diuril. Merck, Sharpe & Dohme
** Chymar. Armour

main difficult to classify the atrophies accurately as to cause. The differentiation is not so difficult by histologic examination. It has been shown[21] that a virus infection is characterized by necrosis of the ganglion cells, whereas in the various hereditary atrophies it is not unusual to find intact ganglion cells in retinae which are atrophic and in which all semblance to normal layer organizations has been lost.

Clinical Signs

11:48   The *subjective symptoms* of hereditary progressive retinal atrophy follow a pattern of regularity. The dog is shy and exhibits defective vision at dusk, at night, or in dimly lighted places, bumping into objects and moving with caution. The animal is usually in the finest of health. The owner may note the pupil dilatation and increased tapetal reflectivity so evident when the dog faces reading lights at night. A different form of progressive retinal atrophy, occurring in the Labrador Retriever, is currently under study by Barnett.[30] It differs from the type herein described in regard to the owner's history, ophthalmoscopic appearance and histopathological changes. Essentially it is a central retinal atrophy, but again is progressive and hereditary.

11:49   *Gross and ophthalmoscopic* findings vary from case to case but, generally, are as follows. In the early stages the pupils are dilated a bit and react sluggishly to light stimuli. Usually the fundi, including the optic discs, will appear normal. As loss of vision progresses, to include day vision as well, the dilatation of the pupils becomes more evident and eventually there will be no response to light stimuli at all. In addition, an increased tapetal reflectivity will be noted, the color of the

tapetum appears to change, and the granular beading of the tapetum is lost.

11:50   Changes in the blood vessels then become marked. The large venules and arterioles remain at first, but are reduced in caliber and become paler. The smaller vessels, meanwhile, become fine and thread-like, and eventually disappear entirely. Meanwhile, the optic discs become paler, changing from pinkish gray to various shades of gray. Then the large vessels, too, become thread-like and the venous circles of the discs are lost. The nontapetal fundi lightens and the optic discs become pale white, and hardly any blood supply can be seen in the fundi.

11:51   The dogs are totally blind before these final stages, which may take from several months to several years to manifest themselves. In early cases the degeneration may be more advanced in one eye than in the other, but as the condition progresses both eyes become equally affected.

11:52   As Barnett[17] points out, "the rate of progression of the atrophy varies considerably from individual to individual, although all cases follow the same pattern. Some owners report a rapid deterioration in vision in a matter of a few weeks, whereas in other cases very little deterioration has been seen, even on ophthalmoscopic examination, inasmuch as six to nine months. The degeneration seems more rapid early after its onset, the rate slowing down as the degeneration advances. It must be remembered, however, that the dog becomes so accustomed to its limited sight, that by using its other senses to an increasing extent, the true rate of degeneration may tend to be masked. It appears that in most cases dogs affected early in life progress to blindness more rapidly than do those which show the first signs of atrophy at a later age."

11:53 Often the owner will exclaim that his pet has gone blind "overnight." In these instances peripheral vision has been gradually lost (Fig. 150), but has gone unnoticed by the owner. Then, when the central vision (area centralis) (Par. 11:15) is affected, the dog's ability to see immediate objects is lost and the assumption is made that blindness was sudden. Ophthalmoscopic examination will readily disclose the progressive changes that have ensued.

11:54 *Stages.* The changes in the fundi of the affected eyes have been described in stages.[22] For sake of convenience, I divide the progressive findings into grades one through four.

11:55 *Grade 1.* Pupils semi-dilated and sluggish to response. Increased tapetal reflectivity, some loss of granular beading, small vessels diminished in caliber and peripheral circulation disappearing. Large venules and arterioles two-thirds normal size.

11:56 *Grade 2.* Pupils dilated, little response. Increased tapetal reflectivity, granular beading nearly gone, smaller vessels nearly all gone, major venules and arterioles one-half normal size, discs paler than normal, non-tapetal fundi lighter.

11:57 *Grade 3.* Pupils dilated, little to no response. Increased tapetal reflectivity, granular beading nearly gone or gone, small vessels completely gone, major venules and arterioles one-third normal size, discs pale, non-tapetal fundi lighter (ashen overcast).

11:58 *Grade 4.* Pupils in full dilation and no response. Increased tapetal reflectivity, granular beading gone, all vessels gone except, possibly, at venous circle. Discs ashen white to white. Absolute total blindness.

11:59 Cataract, secondary to retinal atrophy (Par. 10:33) (Plate 10E), will

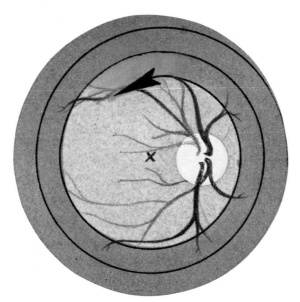

Fig. 150. Mode of progressive loss of vision. Arrow denotes loss from periphery towards the area centralis (X).

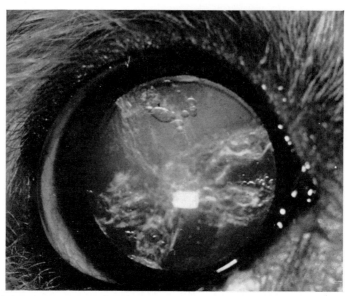

Fig. 151.   Incipient cataract secondary to progressive retinal atrophy. Note vacuoles and streaks extending into the cortex, and dilatation of the pupil. (Courtesy of Keith C. Barnett, Cambridge, England.)

develop in a high percentage of the cases examined. The cataract may be slow or rapid in its development and may affect one eye before the other (Fig. 151). Its formation has been described (Par. 10:34).

11:60   *Treatment.* There is, to date, no known treatment that will materially slow the progress of retinal atrophy or effect a cure. Vitamin A (Par. 3:63) should be prescribed for one month so as to be certain that a deficiency is not responsible for the retinopathy. In some instances of hereditary retinal atrophy it was thought that the changes were slowed down by continuing vitamin A therapy. Once blindness ensues, however, it is useless to continue treatment.

11:61   The sudden blindness associated with a distemper retinopathy may be transient in nature, with partial to full recovery of vision within a few weeks.

Optic Nerve

11:62   *Anatomy.* The optic nerve may be divided into (1) an *intraocular* portion, the head of the optic nerve; (2) an *orbital* portion extending from the eyeball to the optic foramen; and (3) an *intracranial* portion situated between the optic foramen and the chiasm.

11:63   The nerve varies from 1.2 to 2.4 mm in diameter including its sheaths until it enters the eye with the retinal vessels to form the nerve head or disc.[6] This disc can be round, oval, quadrangular, or triangular in shape. It measures about 1 mm in diameter and is slightly below (about 2 mm) and lateral to (about 1 mm) the posterior pole of the globe. It varies in color as well as in shape (Par. 2:59). As the nerve enters the globe the nerve fibers lose their myelin sheath and become transparent.

11:64   The orbital portion of the optic nerve presents a curve, permitting free movement of the eyeball. It is enclosed within a dural sheath continuous with that of the brain, and therefore becomes a compact and enclosed pathway which has no connection with any other neural path until it reaches the cranial cavity. Once outside the orbits, the two optic nerves meet (chiasm) and decussate with each other before distributing to the lateral geniculate bodies (Fig. 3).

Diseases of the Optic Nerve

11:65   *Affections of the optic nerve include:* (1) congenital anomalies; (2) tumors; (3) atrophy; (4) papilledema (choked disc) and, (5) optic neuritis.

11:66   *Congenital anomalies* are commonly observed in the collie breed. A congenital hypoplasia of the optic nerve and retina has been described (Par. 11:19).

11:67   A far more common anomaly was first[23] described as an *excavation of the optic disc* (Plate 11E). Since that time other researchers have employed the terms coloboma of the optic disc or, more recently, congenital posterior ectasia of the sclera.[8]

11:68   *Occurrence.* This problem is believed to be common, with an estimate of 25 per cent of the collies in four blood lines being affected.[8] Most individuals involved will not be presented for an examination unless there is a noticeable visual defect or detachment of the retina or hyphemia occurs. Both sexes are involved and the condition is well distributed throughout the country.

11:69   *Significance.* This disease is important because of its hereditary aspect. Minor defects apparently produce little to no loss of vision, but ectasia of

the posterior sclera, with sclerosis and atrophy of the choroid, may result in degenerative changes in the retina. This anomaly may predispose to retinal detachment, intraocular hemorrhage, (Plate 11F) and glaucoma.

11:70   *Etiology.* The defect consists of arrest of mesodermal development which affects the sclera and the cribriform plate, and is probably related to abnormal differentiation of the optic cup.[8] The exact hereditary pattern is not known.

11:71   *Clinical signs.*[24] The signs depend upon the degree and duration of the involvement of the posterior structures of the eye. Collies may have vision ranging from normal to complete blindness. Breeders may present dogs for examination because of their awareness of the problem within the breed. The age incidence in animals showing signs recognizable to the owner may vary from a few months to five or six years of age.

11:72   Other reasons for presenting a case include: abnormally dilated pupils; prominent fundus reflex; a "membrane inside the eye" (detached retina); intraocular hemorrhage; corneal opacity; and cataract. It has been my experience that, in those cases showing intraocular hemorrhage, the left eye was involved and the blood remained in a fluid state in the anterior chamber, diminishing in amount from time to time, only to return.[23]

11:73   The *ophthalmoscopic findings* vary from case to case. The lesion common to all eyes is an enlargement and excavation of the optic disc. The disc may appear to be from two to five times its normal size. The vessels drop off the edge of the excavation and may require a lens of minus 8 to minus 20 diopters to be brought into focus as they cross the floor of the disc. In others, a part of the disc will look normal while one edge will show a deep hole or a pale avascular area immediately adjacent to it. There may be a posterior bulging of the sclera at the inferonasal or temporal edge of the disc. Other eyes may take on a gray ground glass appearance in this same area and contain only a few retinal vessels with no sign of underlying choroid. The blood vessels usually show increased tortuosity as they approach the disc. Saunders[25] believes that some of the tortuosity of the vessels is due to the fact that the optic nerve enters the eye at a more acute angle than normal because the eyes are rotated away from the proper axis and getting too close to the midline.

11:74　　Changes in the color of the tapetal portion of the fundus are frequently observed. The yellow-green reflex is replaced by an orange-red color, and the underlying choroidal vessels, which are normally invisible above the disc, can be seen. Some dogs show some degree of normal tapetal coloration, while others show none. Examination of many normal collies may prove this finding to have no significance other than it occurs in certain families of dogs.

11:75　　Retinal detachments may be seen in a small percentage of affected animals. The most striking of these is the total serous detachment which prevents visualization of the disc and appears as a tremulous pink membrane which is thrown into folds which wave and change position as the eye moves (Par. 11:37).

11:76　　Some eyes in the advanced stages of the condition show degrees of retinal degeneration (Par. 11:38), and

small (1 to 3 mm) gray patches in the retina (cysts?). These animals have marked loss of vision.

11:77　　A most significant clinical finding is a small eye. Collie breeders have become more and more conscious of the fact that dogs cannot win in shows unless they have small eyes with almond-shaped lid aperture. Large-eyed collies have been deemed undesirable and are disappearing from the scene. It seems more than coincidental that the incidence of this condition has increased along with the trend of breeding for a small eye. Since microphthalmos is known to be associated with coloboma of the disc, choroid and retina, there is a good basis for stressing the importance of eye size. Corneal opacities and congenital cataract have been seen in affected pups.

11:78　　*Tumors* of the optic nerve are rare, being derived from the nerve sheaths (meningioma) and from the glial framework (glioma). Williams *et al.*[26] reported on a retrobulbar glioma of the optic nerve which developed along the course of the left optic nerve to the optic chiasm and then along the course of the right optic nerve. I encountered a confirmed meningioma in a male, eleven-year-old collie (Fig. 152A). He had been blind for one month and the left eye exhibited the classic findings of an advanced retrobulbar tumor (Par. 8:26). In addition, the retina appeared detached. The pupil of the right eye was dilated and responded slowly to light stimuli. On necropsy, a fairly round, firm tumor of the optic nerve was found tightly adhered to the posterior axis of the globe (Fig. 152B). It had started to necrotize.

11:79　　Tumors of the optic nerve produce early loss of vision and exophthalmos (Par. 8:26). This condition is unilateral, and must be distinguished from other orbital inflammatory processes and causes of unilateral exophthalmos (Par. 8:15). Treatment consists in removal of the growth by the Kroenlein operation (Par. 8:29) or by exenteration of the orbit (Par. 8:42).

11:80   *Atrophy* is the end result of destructive disease involving the optic nerves.[27] Optic atrophy is caused by:

direct pressure from neoplasia; glaucoma chorioretinitis; intracranial hemorrhage; avitaminosis A; following optic neuritis; toxic conditions involving the optic pathway; and, it is associated with progressive retinal atrophy (Fig. 153). Sometimes degenerative processes of unknown cause result in progressive atrophy.

11:81   McGrath[28] has observed unilateral optic atrophy in the dog in four

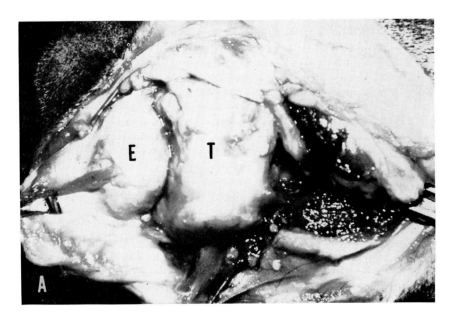

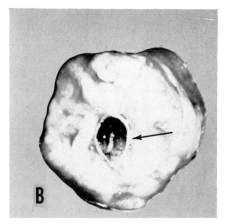

Fig. 152.   A. Necropsy view of retrobulbar meningioma. E. Eyeball. T. Tumor. B. Tumor attached to a portion of the posterior sclera and to the optic nerve.

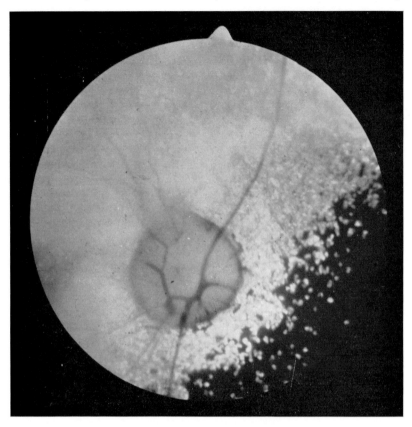

Fig. 153. Optic disc atrophy associated with progressive retinal atrophy. Note diminution in size and number of retinal vessels. (Courtesy of Keith C. Barnett, Cambridge, England).

cases, three in which the pathology (a cyst or tumor) compressed the optic nerve within the orbital fossa (Fig. 154); and one case in which a middle fossa meningioma had compressed the right optic nerve within the cranial cavity.

11:82 We have observed optic atrophy as an end result of all the aforementioned causes, including two cases of poisoning. In one, inhalation of exterminator gas was believed responsible and, in the second, dipping in a "lye" solution resulted in incoordination and loss of vision.

11:83 *Ophthalmoscopic signs* of optic atrophy vary and depend upon the cause and the stage. The disc is pale gray to chalk white and may be reduced in size. Its margins may be sharply defined or irregular. The blood vessels normally present are few in number or gone altogether. Pigment migration from the surrounding structures causes the outline to be blurred and indistinct.

11:84 *Prognosis.* Since atrophy of the nerve fibers has involved a great part of the optic nerve before a dog is presented and a diagnosis is made, the probability of restoration of function is poor. However, if some central vision remains, removal of the cause of the disease may preserve that vision.

11:85 *Treatment* consists in attempting to control the cause. Little can be done for the atrophy itself.

11:86   *Papilledema* (choked disc) is a swelling or edema of the optic nerve head resulting from increased intracranial pressure. In man, approximately 50 per cent of patients with brain tumor exhibit this lesion. Routine fundic examinations have been carried out in many dogs with verified brain tumors, intracranial trauma, optic neuritis which occurred in association with viral encephalitis, and other lesions producing increased intracranial pressure. To date, true clinical examples of papilledema

have been encountered rarely in the dog.[28]

11:87   I encountered a pronounced papilledema in a boxer which later was euthanized and found to have a retrobulbar rhabdomyosarcoma (Par. 8:27). When initially presented, clinical signs included a moderate exophthalmos and conjunctival chemosis. The well-developed choked disc showed an elevation of 6 diopters over the surrounding area (Par. 2:50).

11:88   A second case involved a collie which suddenly lost vision. Both pupils were dilated with no response

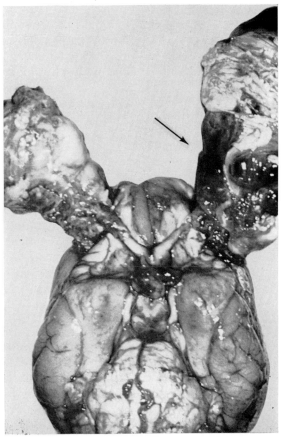

Fig. 154. Postorbital neurogenic sarcoma in a nine-year-old male Boxer. The tumor produced unilateral atrophy by compression. Note exophthalmic deviation of the globe. (Courtesy of Dr. John T. McGrath, Philadelphia, Pa.)

to light stimuli. Edema of the discs appeared to involve the surrounding retina (neuroretinitis) (Plate 11G), and small hemorrhages or aneurysms were noted in the vessels as they emerged from the disc. Treatment with steroids, vitamin B₁₂, and Diuril* effected considerable improvement in vision. Some of the edema left the discs, but vision was lost again within a few months. At this writing the condition remains unchanged, with the cause undetermined.

11:89   *Optic neuritis* (papillitis) is a broad term denoting inflammation, degeneration or demyelinization of the optic nerve. The term "optic neuritis" also includes retrobulbar neuritis, a form in which the nerve is affected posteriorly so that there are no visible ophthalmoscopic changes of the nerve head.

11:90   It is my opinion that a form of retrobulbar neuritis is not uncommon to the dog. We encounter cases exhibiting a sudden loss of vision and dilated pupils, but with an absence of ophthalmoscopic findings (Par. 11:92). Acute retrobulbar neuritis tends to run its course in a period of from one to six weeks. Response to treatment within two weeks of onset is a good sign. There may be partial to complete return of vision, but relapses occur, with total blindness ensuing.

11:91   *Treatment.* Administration of repositol B₁₂ (1000 mg) at four-day intervals, ACTH every second day, prednisone tablets and vitamin A is suggested. If there is no response to this therapy within two weeks, it is usually useless to continue.

Amaurosis

11:92   Amaurosis is a term used to describe blindness for which the cause

* Diuril, Merck, Sharpe & Dohme.

is unknown. A tentative diagnosis of amaurosis is often made when blindness suddenly occurs in an apparently healthy dog in which there is no associated clinical signs or ophthalmoscopic findings. Later it is sometimes possible to discover the cause. As other neurological findings become evident, or, by virtue of a necropsy, a brain tumor, for example, may be elicited as the cause. Response to the treatment for retrobulbar neuritis is suggestive that this condition was responsible for the amaurosis. Vitamin A deficiency resulting in amaurosis will respond quickly to this medication. But, in the majority of instances the true cause of amaurosis remains unknown.

11:93   Neuro-ophthalmology is a most complex subject. Even with a precise knowledge of the neuroanatomy and neurophysiology of the visual pathways, it would be impossible for a veterinary clinician to evaluate visual field defects in his patients without the aid of the functional tests, *i.e.*, perimetry, so useful in man.

11:94   *Treatment.* Determination of the cause by careful evaluation of the history, clinical signs, and ophthalmoscopic findings, and, repeated examinations of the patient, may be necessary if the diagnosis of amaurosis is to be changed to a more positive one. In the interim, however, the treatment suggested for retrobulbar neuritis (Par. 11:91) may be started.

11:95   *Amblyopia* is a reduction in visual acuity, not dependent upon any visible changes in the eye. This partial loss of vision may be transient in nature and is usually accompanied by loss of co-ordination. It is caused by drug, chemical, or disease intoxication.

11:96   *Blindness* in dogs is conveniently divided into four main groups:[29] (1) those due to defects in the optical system of the eye, such as corneal, lens, or vitreal opacities; (2) those due to disturbances of the retina; (3) those relating to the optic pathways between the retina and the brain; and, (4) disorders of the perception areas of the brain itself (Fig. 3).

References

1. Adler, Francis H.: *Physiology of the Eye,* 2nd ed., St. Louis, The C. V. Mosby Co., p. 219–225, 1953.
2. Fine, Ben S. and Tousimis, A. J.: The Structure of the Vitreous Body and the Suspensory Ligaments of the Lens, Arch. Ophth., *65,* 95–110, 1961.
3. Rodman, H. I., Johnson, F. B., and Zimmerman, L. E.: New Histopathological and Histochemical Observations Concerning Asteroid Hyalitis, Arch. Ophth., *66,* 552–563, 1961.
4. Magrane, William G.: Ocular Physiology–Clinical Application, No. Am. Vet., *36,* 564, 1955.
5. Rubin, Lionel F.: Asteroid Hyalosis in the Dog, Am. J. Vet. Res., *24,* 1256–1262, 1963.
6. Prince, Jack H., Diesem, Charles D., Eglitis, Irma, and Ruskill, Gordon, L.: *Anatomy and Histology of the Eye and Orbit in Domestic Animals,* Springfield, Charles C Thomas, 1960.
7. Saunders, Leon Z.: Congenital Optic Nerve Hypoplasia in Collie Dogs, Cornell Vet., *62,* 67–80, 1952.
8. Roberts, Seymour, R.: Congenital Posterior Ectasia of the Sclera in Collie Dogs, Am. J. Ophth., *50,* 451–465, 1960.
9. Rubin, Lionel F.: Hereditary Retinal Detachment in Bedlington Terriers, Sm. Am. Clinician, *3,* 387–389, 1963.
10. Rubin, Lionel F.: Atypical Coloboma of the Choroid in a Dog, J.A.V.M.A., *143,* 841–842, 1963.
11. Catcott, Earl J.: Ophthalmoscopy in Canine Practice, J.A.V.M.A., *121,* 35–37, 1952.
12. Roberts, Seymour R.: Detachment of the Retina in Animals, J.A.V.M.A., *135,* 423–431, 1959.
13. Grice, H. C. and Hutchison, J. A.: Retinoblastoma in a Dog, J.A.V.M.A., *136,* 444–446, 1960.
14. Magnusson, H.: Arch. Vergl. Ophth., *2,* 147, 1911.
15. Hodgman, F. S. J., Parry, H. B., Rasbridge, W. J. and Steel, J. D.: Progressive Retinal Atrophy in Dogs, Vet. Rec., *61,* 185, 1949.
16. Schnelle, Gerald B.: Progressive Retinal Atrophy in a Dog, J.A.V.M.A., *121,* 177–178, 1952.
17. Barnett, K. C.: Hereditary Retinal Atrophy in the Poodle, Vet. Rec., *74,* 672–675, 1962.
18. Magrane, William G.: Progressive Retinal Atrophy and Associated Blindness: Breed Incidence, No. Am. Vet., *36,* 743–746, 1955.
19. Parry, H. B.: Degenerations of the Dog Retina, Brit. J. Ophth., *38,* 295–309, 1954.
20. Parry, H. B.: Generalized Progressive Atrophy of Uncertain Etiology, Brit. J. Ophth., *38,* 545, 1954.
21. Jubb, K. U., Saunders, Leon Z., and Coates, H. U.: The Intraocular Lesions of Canine Distemper, J. Comp. Path. & Ther., *67,* 21–29, 1957.
22. Smythe, R. H.: *Veterinary Ophthalmology,* London, Baillière Tindall & Cox, p. 327, 1956.
23. Magrane, William G.: Congenital Anomaly of the Optic Disc in Collies, No. Am. Vet., *34,* 646, 1953.
24. Report—Comm. on Ophth. of the Am. An. Hosp. Assoc., 1960.
25. Saunders, Leon Z.: The Clinical Appearance and Pathology of Some Congenital Ocular Defects in Collie Dogs, Proc. Am. Soc. Vet. Ophth., 1960.
26. Williams, J. O., Garlick, E. C., Beard, D. C.: Glioma of the Optic Nerve of a Dog J.A.V.M.A., *138,* 377–378, 1961.
27. Leinfelder, P. J.: Outline of Neuro-ophthalmology. Home Study Course, Am. Ac. Ophth. & Otol., 1950.
28. McGrath, John T.: *Neurologic Examination of the Dog,* 2nd Ed. Philadelphia, Lea & Febiger, p. 29, 1960.
29. Parry, H. B.: Vet. Rec., *63,* 323, 1951.
30. Barnett, K. C.: Canine Retinopathies, Thesis in press.

Chapter 12

THE OCULAR MANIFESTATIONS OF SYSTEMIC DISEASE

"The light of the body is the eye."
Matthew 6:22

12:1 Ophthalmology should be considered as an integral part of internal medicine. The ocular condition often appears early in the course of a systemic disease and may be important to the diagnosis and prognosis. The ocular symptoms occurring with systemic affections are discussed more fully in the preceding chapters. Little has been written for the veterinary literature on the subject for this chapter. Considerable research and clinical observation is needed to correlate more accurately eye findings and diseases of the dog.

Diseases of the Blood

12:2 *Anemia* gives rise to pale pink conjunctivae and a pearly white sclerae.

The retinal vessels are more pale than normal and, depending upon the cause, retinal hemorrhages are occasionally found.

12:3 *Lipemia.* The anterior chambers are partially to fully filled with a very fluid milky exudate. When ophthalmoscopy is possible, the blood of the retinal vessels appears "creamy," *i.e.,* like light tomato juice. The "silver wire" reflection (Par. 2:58) from the vessels in the non-tapetal fundus is absent.

12:4 A paracentesis (Par. 6:143) will temporarily clear the anterior chamber, but the secondary aqueous which fills the chamber is also milky. Thyroid therapy and a low fat diet will result in permanent clearing within a week.

12:5 *Purpura* may be accompanied

by petechial hemorrhages beneath the conjunctiva, in the retina, and in the skin of the lids.

Diseases of the Digestive System

12:6 *Teeth.* A septic mouth from infected teeth may predispose to conjunctival congestion and iritis (Par. 7:28).

12:7 *Liver.* Diseases of the liver may cause jaundice, a yellowish discoloration of the sclera and of the conjunctiva.

12:8 *Pancreas.* In chronic pancreatitis interference with the digestion of fat may lead to a deficiency of vitamin A. This, in turn, can result in a loss of vision. Fortunately this type of blindness is reversible. If diagnosed in time, daily administration of vitamin A (Par. 3:63) will correct the condition.

Diseases of the Kidneys

12:9 *Nephritis* may present ocular manifestations in the late stages. In uremia retinal hemorrhages are not uncommon (Par. 11:24) and are an indication that death is imminent. These hemorrhages vary in size and shape, are usually seen near the vessels, and are flame-shaped (superficial) or small and round (deeper layers). Conjunctival congestion and discharges are also indicative of the toxic state of the animal.

Diseases of the Muscles

12:10 *Eosinophilic myositis* (Par. 8: 20) produces striking ocular symptoms. Exophthalmos, edema of the lids, conjunctival chemosis, and hypertrophy and protrusion of the membrane nictitans can be expected in the acute form (Plate 8B).

12:11 *Atrophy* of the muscles around the eye and of the postorbital fat following an attack of eosinophilic myositis

will result in an enophthalmos of the globe (Par. 8:32) (Plate 8D).

Diseases of the Endocrine Glands and Metabolic Disorders

12:12 *Pituitary.* Neoplasm of the pituitary gland causes impairment of vision of various degrees and an eventual partial or complete atrophy of the optic nerve. This amaurosis (Par. 11: 92), of course, remains unsolved until confirmed on necropsy. McGrath[1] has encountered pituitary adenocarcinomas in which amaurosis was initially noted.

12:13 *Dysproteinemia.* Darraspen and Lescure[2] report a case of a dog with an endocular hemorrhage and a concurrent dysproteinemia.

12:14 *Diabetes.* The common ocular complication of diabetes in the dog is cataract (Par. 10:29). The retinopathy associated with diabetes in man has not been commonly observed in the dog. The characteristic diabetic retinopathy of man includes the findings of: capillary microaneurysms; dot and blot hemorrhages; retinal and vitreous hemorrhage; and, retinal detachment.

12:15 Catcott[3] was unable to detect fundic changes in a series of dogs subjected to experimental diabetes. His observation period, however, was over a short period of time. Gross retinal lesions do not appear in diabetic humans until after a considerable time lapse. Recently capillary aneurysms have been clearly demonstrated by Patz and Maumenee[4] in a spontaneously diabetic dog. Engerman and Bloodworth[5] have produced experimental diabetic retinopathy in dogs. Retinae of ten dogs were studied histologically after nine to sixty-nine months of alloxan or metasomatropin diabetes. Either type of diabetes was found to result in a retinopathy comparable to that of human diabetes mellitus. The retinopathy occurred in each of three dogs that had been diabetic over four years. The evidence indicated that diabetic retinopathy is dependent to a lesser extent on the cause of diabetes than on its duration, and is a result not of a genetic disorder but of metabolic alterations initiated by deficiency of insulin.

Diseases of the Ear, Nose, Throat and Accessory Sinuses

12:16 *Ear.* Nystagmus is common in affections of the labyrinth and vestibular pathways. A chronic purulent conjunctivitis may be associated with purulent otitis (Par. 5:41).

12:17 *Nose and Throat.* The communication between the nose and the conjunctival sac by means of the lacrimal duct explains the occurrence of ocular symptoms as a result of nasal disease. In seasonal allergy there is often a conjunctival congestion or acute catarrhal conjunctivitis with marked lacrimation. Conjunctivitis may be a complication of chronic rhinitis. The lacrimal duct may be the means of conveying infective material from the nose to the conjunctival sac.

12:18 *Throat.* The tonsils merit consideration as a focus of infection in inflammations and infections of the eyes. Chronically infected tonsils must be regarded as a likely source for endogenous infection. Iritis and uveitis may occur as a manifestation of tonsillar infection (Par. 7:28).

12:19 *Sinus* disease may be responsible for ocular symptoms which include orbital cellulitis (Par. 8:17) (Plate 8A); conjunctivitis; and, iritis with deep keratitis in a small percentage of cases.

Diseases of the Nervous System

12:20 *Nystagmus.* Congenital nystagmus should probably be regarded as the result, or manifestation, of some other congenital or hereditary condition.[6] It is sometimes called visual nystagmus and results from conditions causing great loss of vision in both eyes, before or at the time of birth. In man, any of the ocular conditions such as congenital cataracts, anomalies of the retina or choroid, and congenital opacities on the cornea might produce so-called congenital nystagmus.

12:21 We have seen nystagmus associated with microphthalmia, a fixed pupil, divergent strabismus and detachment of the retina. A visual nystagmus may be associated with any of the congenital anomalies of the fundus previously described (Par. 11:19–11:21).

12:22 *Horner's syndrome* is characterized by unilateral miosis, ptosis, and enophthalmos. It is caused most frequently by lesions producing paralysis of the cervical sympathetic portion of the autonomic nervous system and lesions of the hypothalamus. McGrath[7] has observed the syndrome with tumors of the anterior mediastinum, cervical cord lesions (especially tumors), and tumors of the hypothalamus.

Infectious and Mycotic Diseases

12:23 *Distemper.* A variable degree of conjunctivitis is to be expected in nearly every case of distemper. Corneal ulceration (Par. 6:91) and/or keratitis sicca (Par. 6:57) are less frequent manifestations.

12:24 Transient or permanent blindness occurs in still fewer instances (Par. 11:46). Intraocular lesions may be present concurrently with or in the absence of brain lesions.[8] Varying degrees of retinal atrophy has been found on histologic examination. Gross findings include dilatation of the pupil, but an essentially normal appearing fundus (Par. 11:46).

12:25 *Hepatitis.* A serous conjunctivitis may be present, but in the mild form, ocular manifestations are seldom apparent. A corneal opacity of one or both eyes may appear after the acute illness has subsided (Par. 7:29). These opacities are usually transitory.

12:26 *Leptospirosis.* Inflammation of the conjunctiva and a catarrhal to crusty discharge can be expected. In the icterohemorrhagiae form a jaundiced sclera and petechial hemorrhages beneath the conjunctiva are the usual findings.

12:27 *Toxoplasmosis* of man is known to be responsible for uveitis and chorioretinitis. Sufficient evidence has been accumulated to indicate that some relationship may exist between animal and human toxoplasmosis, although evidence of communicability is lacking.[9] Heeley[10] believes that this organism may be involved in some of our more obscure clinical problems (Par. 7:51). Barron and Saunders[12] have found toxoplasma organisms in the enucleated eye of a dog. The associated pathologic changes were retinitis, iridocyclitis, and optic neuritis.

12:28 Undoubtedly an occasional case of uveitis with a subsequent chorioretinitis in the dog can be attributed to toxoplasmosis. In general, however, fewer ocular manifestations will be found in dogs infected with toxoplasma than in a like number in man.[11] In cases of recurrent uveitis is has been my practice to confirm or eliminate toxoplasma as a source through use of the Sabin-Feldman dye test.

12:29 *Rabies.* Possible findings in this disease include: reddened conjunctiva; mucopurulent exudate; anisocoria (uneven pupils); divergent or convergent strabismus; and a membrane nictitans protruding over the globe.

12:30 *Tetanus.* The membrane nictitans is usually prominent and is seen to flick over the eyes. The pupils are miotic.

12:31 *Septicemia* alone may produce manifestations in almost any of the structures of the eye. The more common are those of the conjunctiva (discharge, petechial hemorrhages). A generalized septicemia can lead to involvement of the uveal tract (iridocyclitis with hypopyon) or an endophthalmitis and ultimate loss of the eyeball (Par. 7:53).

12:32 *Coccidioidomycosis* is known to produce severe corneal and conjunctival involvement. Cello[13] has demonstrated the natural occurrence of a granulomatous uveitis in dogs with disseminated coccidioidomycosis and points out that a true evaluation of the incidence of this condition can only be obtained from careful examination of the eye by veterinarians practicing in areas where the disease is endemic.

12:33 *Blastomycosis* may produce eye discharges and loss of vision, probably stemming from a uveitis.[14]

12:34 *Cryptococcosis* has been reported as being the cause of blindness in the dog.[15, 16] Full pupil dilatation was observed in those cases reported.

Malignancies

12:35 *Malignant Lymphoma* (lymphosarcoma). (Plate 6H and Fig. 155). The ocular changes in malignant lymphoma of dogs are striking. These changes

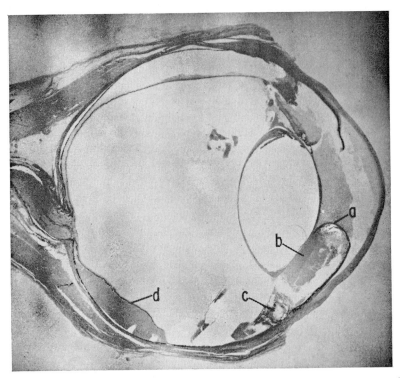

Fig. 155.   Canine malignant lymphoma. Section of eye showing iris bombé and atrophic iris (*a*), hemorrhage in posterior chamber (*b*), atrophy of ciliary body (*c*), subretinal hemorrhage (*d*). (Cello and Hutcherson, courtesy of Cornell Veterinarian.)

are significant in that they occur more frequently than has been supposed, and they may, on occasion, precede the actual systemic symptoms of the disease.

12:36   Cello and Hutcherson[17] summarize the most important changes found in the various parts of the globe. Conjunctivitis ranges in severity from a mild inflammation with hyperemia, chemosis, and scanty mucous discharge to a severe purulent discharge with thickening and induration of the tissue. Changes in the cornea include edema, vascularization, keratic precipitates, and intrastromal hemorrhage. Ulcerative keratitis is a common finding in the final stages of the disease and usually appears after the cornea has undergone one or more of the other corneal

changes. A dense white band around the limbal margin of the cornea may be noted. This infiltrate is an evasion of tumor cells.

12:37   Spontaneous hemorrhage into the anterior chamber (hyphema) is a frequent gross sign of tumor involvement. Uveitis and a hazy ocular media is part of the picture. This makes ophthalmoscopy difficult, if not impossible, in some cases. When the fundus can be viewed, a retinopathy with superficial flame-shaped and deep round hemorrhages may be evident.

12:38   Glaucoma is to be expected as a secondary complication of the later stages.[18] Tumor involvement of the iris, ciliary body and retina will, in turn, produce the rise in tension.

12:39 In general, examination of the eye will not be helpful in detecting early cases of malignant lymphoma, since by the time the ocular changes occur, the more common systemic symptoms are evident. This is not always true, however. I have examined eyes in which the neoplastic infiltration of the cornea had been mistaken clinically for an obscure keratitis, and others in which the tumor tissue had partially filled the anterior chamber. Further examination of the patient then revealed the beginning lymph node enlargement.

12:40 *Intracranial Tumors.* Interruption of the optic pathways in association with neoplasia will produce partial to total loss of vision of one or both eyes. This amaurosis (Par. 11:92) may precede certain specific neurologic signs and symptoms which are then suggestive of an intracranial malignancy.

12:41 *Retrobulbar Tumors* (Par. 8: 25) (Plate 8E and F). Depending upon the stage of development, one or all of these ocular manifestations are present. Exophthalmos, globe deviation, diminished movement; prominent hypertrophied membrane nictitans; pupil dilated and/or eccentric; exposure keratitis; and, blindness.

12:42 *Secondary Intraocular Tumors.* These tumors occur by hematogenous metastasis from the internal organs. They also occur from the orbit, conjunctiva, or cornea via the optic nerve or cornea.[19] It is believed that the examination of the eye in cases of generalized neoplasia in animals will reveal that intraocular metastasis are far from rare.

Parasitism

12:43 *Hookworm.* A severe hookworm infestation will give rise to a pale conjunctivae and pearly white sclera (anemia). An accompanying mucopurulent conjunctival discharge can be expected.

12:44 *Heartworm.* The filarial worm has been observed in the anterior chamber on several occasions. An increase in lacrimation and some corneal hazing accompanies this unusual condition.

12:45 *Mange.* Demodex or sarcoptic mange can produce a blepharitis (Par. 4:62).

Deficiencies

12:46 *Vitamin A.* The principal ocular manifestations of an avitaminosis A are erosion of corneal tissue (keratomalacia) (Par. 6:92) (Plate 5D) and loss of vision. I have examined blind puppies and adult dogs that were being fed diets deficient in vitamin A. In some instances the pupil response was good and, from all appearances, the fundi was still unaffected. In others, pupillary response was sluggish and retinal degeneration was in evidence. Correction of the diet and a therapeutic regimen of vitamin A resulted in return of vision (Par. 3:58).

12:47 *Riboflavin* (B$_2$) deficiency is characterized by superficial vascularization with a possible ulceration and subsequent opacity of the cornea.

Poisonings and Intoxications

12:48 Drug and chemical poisonings may produce eye manifestations. These may develop as the direct result of an acute or chronic intoxication and include contraction or dilatation of the pupils, retinal hemorrhages, amblyopia (Par. 11:95) and cataract.

References

1. McGrath, John T.: Personal Communication, 1954.

2. Darraspen, E. and Lescure, F.: A Propos d'un cas d'hémorragie endoculaire Relation possible avec une dysprotéinémie, Revue de Medecine Veterinaire, *111,* 275, 1960.

3. Catcott, Earl J.: Ophthalmoscopy in Canine Practice, J.A.V.M.A., *121,* 37, 1952.

4. Patz, A. and Maumenee, A. E.: Studies on Diabetic Retinopathy, 1. Retinopathy in Dog with Spontaneous Diabetes Mellitus, Am. J. Ophth., *54,* 532–541, 1962.

5. Engerman, R. L. and Bloodworth, J. M. B.: Experimental Diabetic Retinopathy in Dogs, Arch. Ophth., *73,* 205–210, 1965.

6. Tassman, I. S.: *The Eye Manifestations of Internal Diseases,* 3rd, St. Louis, The C. V. Mosby Co., p. 286, 1951.

7. McGrath, John T.: *Neurologic Examination of the Dog,* Philadelphia, Lea & Febiger, p. 26, 1956.

8. Jubb, K. V., Saunders, Leon Z. and Coates, Helen V.: The Intraocular Lesions of Canine Distemper, J. Comp. Path. & Ther., *67,* 21–29, 1957.

9. Cole, Clarence R., et al: Toxoplasmosis III. Study of Families Exposed to Their Toxoplasma-Infected Pet Dogs, A.M.A. Arch. Int. Med., *92,* 308–313, 1953.

10. Heeley, D. M.: Toxoplasmosis, J. Sm. An. Pract., *4,* 435–446, 1963.

11. Cole, Clarence R.: Personal Communication, 1954.

12. Barron, Von C. N. and Saunders, Leon Z.: Ein Fall von intraokulärer Toxoplasmose beim Hund, Schweizer Archiv für Tierheilkunde, *101,* 7, 1959.

13. Cello, Robert M.: Ocular Manifestations of Coccidioidomycosis in a Dog, Arch. Ophth., *64,* 897–903, 1960.

14. Selby, Lloyd A., et al: Canine Blastomycosis, Sm. An. Clinician, *59,* 1221–1228, 1964.

15. *Canine Medicine,* 2nd ed., Santa Barbara, American Veterinary Publications, Inc., p. 636, 1959.

16. Trautwein, G. and Nielsen, S. W.: Cryptococcosis in 2 Cats, a Dog, and a Mink, J.A.V.M.A., *140,* 438, 1962.

17. Cello, Robert M. and Hutcherson, Brian: Ocular Changes in Malignant Lymphoma, Cornell Vet., *52,* 492–523, 1962.

18. Saunders, Leon Z. and Barron, Von C. N.: Intraocular Tumors in Animals: IV. Lymphosarcoma, Brit. Vet. J., *120,* 25–35, 1964.

19. Barron, Von C. N., Saunders, Leon Z. and Jebb, K. V.: Intraocular Tumors in Animals. III. Secondary Intraocular Tumors, Am. J. Vet. Res., *24,* 835–853, 1963.

Appendix 1

Breed Predisposition to Conditions of the Eye

Afghan hound
Juvenile cataract

Basset hound
Secondary glaucoma (subluxated lens)

Beagle
Progressive retinal atrophy

Bedlington terrier
Distichiasis
Lacrimal duct atresia
Retinal detachment

Blood hound
Ectropian

Boston terrier
Hypertrophy of the nictitans gland
Juvenile cataract

Boxer
Recurrent corneal erosion

Bulldog (English)
Ectropion
Entropion

Cairn terrier
Secondary glaucoma (subluxated lens)

Chesapeake Bay retriever
Progressive retinal atrophy
Entropion

Chihauhua
Keratitis sicca
Secondary glaucoma (subluxated lens)

Chow Chow
Narrow palpebral fissure
Entropion

Cocker spaniel
Ectropion
Hypertrophy of the nictitans gland
Acute congestive primary glaucoma
Secondary glaucoma (subluxated lens)
Juvenile cataract
Progressive retinal atrophy

Collie
Microphthalmos
Retinal detachment
Progressive retinal atrophy
Optic nerve hypoplasia
Excavation of optic disc (scleral ectasia)

English setter
Progressive retinal atrophy

Fox terrier, smooth
Secondary glaucoma (subluxated lens)

Fox terrier, wire-haired
Secondary glaucoma (subluxated lens)
Juvenile cataract

German shepherd
Pannus

Golden retriever
Progressive retinal atrophy
Entropion

Gordon setter
Progressive retinal atrophy

Great Dane
Eversion of membrane nictitans

Irish setter
Progressive retinal atrophy

Kerry blue terrier
Narrow palpebral fissure
Entropion

Labrador retriever
Progressive retinal atrophy
Entropion

Manchester terrier
Secondary glaucoma (subluxated
lens)

Miniature pincher
Keratitis sicca

Norwegian Elkhound
Progressive retinal atrophy

Pekingese
Distichiasis
Pigmentary keratitis
Virulent corneal ulceration

Pointer
Progressive retinal atrophy

Pomeranian
Epiphora

Poodle
Distichiasis
Lacrimal duct atresia
Epiphora
Microphthalmos
Juvenile cataract
Progressive retinal atrophy

Pug
Pigmentary keratitis

Rottweiler
Entropion

Saint Bernard
Entropion
Ectropion
Eversion membrane nictitans

Sealyham terrier
Lacrimal duct atresia
Secondary glaucoma (subluxated
lens)

Springer spaniel
Progressive retinal atrophy

Schnauzer, miniature
Microphthalmos
Juvenile cataract

Toy terrier
Secondary glaucoma (subluxated
lens)

Weimariner
Eversion membrane nictitans

Welsh corgi
Secondary glaucoma (subluxated
lens)

Yorkshire terrier
Keratitis sicca

Appendix 2

Uses of Adrenal Steroids in Eye Diseases[*]

Steroids have little permanent effect on hypersensitive reactions in the eye. They reduce inflammatory reaction but when withdrawn, the ocular relapse is as severe as if therapy had not been instituted.

Steroids have the effect of restoring an abnormally increased capillary permeability to normal.

Prior or simultaneous administration of a steroid will reduce the penetration of an antibiotic into an eye.

Steroids and ACTH are capable of profoundly modifying the issue reaction to infection. When this reaction is so violent as to be harmful, the anti-inflammatory reaction of the steroids can be useful. At the same time, unless antibiotic chemotherapy is employed, the steroid may mask the progress of the infecting agent.

Newer compounds. It appears that the effects are similar to those of the older compounds except they may be obtained at lower dosage levels.

Evaluation of therapy with steroids in eye diseases depends on the following factors:

1. Accurate diagnosis. It is desirable to know if the disease is due to an in-

fection, allergy, circulatory disturbance, or injury.

2. Stage of disease. Severe eye inflammations which have existed for some time respond to a lesser degree than do those which have been present for a short period. On the other hand, such a disease as optic neuritis which has been active for six weeks might be expected to show spontaneous improvement at about this time; therefore, the results of therapy would be difficult to evaluate.

3. Course of disease. In evaluating the results of therapy one must keep in mind that a reasonable number of eye diseases have a predictable course. Many self-limiting conditions should not be treated. Other self-limiting conditions respond more rapidly to steroid therapy than to other methods of treatment. Still other diseases might have a prolonged course but respond well to steroid therapy and should be treated energetically.

4. Nature and site of lesion. The position of the lesion in the eye and surrounding structures determines the type of therapy to be given. Severe anterior ocular inflammation probably should be treated with topical as well as oral or intravenous corticosteroid therapy. Less severe inflammation can be treated by topical therapy (drops, ointment, or subconjunctival injection). Posterior ocular disease should be treated by oral or intravenous therapy, since topically

[*] Abstracted from: Brown, J., Pearson, C. M. (Eds.): *Clinical Uses of Adrenal Steroids,* New York, McGraw-Hill Book Co., Inc., p. 186–222, 1962.

233

applied drugs do not penetrate to the posterior eye.

Failure of an intraocular inflammation to respond to local or systemic corticosteroid therapy may occur for several reasons:

1. The inflammation is of microbial origin, and the corticosteroid has facilitated dissemination of the organisms.

2. Therapy has been instituted too late.

3. Inadequate dosage. Some severe inflammations require large initial doses.

4. Lack of utilization of all routes of therapy—systemic, topical, and subjunctival injection—for conditions in which all three are indicated, as in some types of conjunctival, corneal, and anterior segment inflammation.

Occasionally a patient responds well to one corticosteroid and poorly to another; the reason for this is obscure, but the authors have seen several such instances. If failure occurs, one should consider exchanging the steroid preparation being used for another.

Contraindications: Bacterial corneal infections and ulceration should not be treated with corticosteroids alone, or in combination with antibiotics, because of the danger of superinfection with other bacteria or the development of a fungus infection. Viral corneal infections should not be treated with any type of corticosteroid even though this therapy seems to produce relief from pain and inflammation.

Index